"WHAT KIND OF REDUCING DIET SHOULD I CHOOSE?"

is a question which plagues many of us. There are so many different diets on the market that it is often difficult to pick the good from the bad. As Victor Lindlahr points out, "To befuddle fatties with reducing diets which cannot possibly work has become a major occupation."

EAT AND REDUCE is a diet book that works! Its success can be measured by the fact that it has already had twenty printings in various editions.*

Why is this book so effective? The reason is simply that although only one person in a thousand likes being overweight, only one in a hundred will go on a starvation diet to shave off those extra pounds.

EAT AND REDUCE is a new kind of diet book! It won't limit you to salads and vegetables. With Victor H. Lindlahr's Low Carbohydrate diet you can lose seven pounds in a week while still eating three square meals a day.

*To see what readers say about this book, please turn to the last page.

EAT—
and Reduce!

Victor H. Lindlahr

PERMABOOKS • *New York, N.Y.*

EAT—AND REDUCE!

Prentice-Hall edition published December, 1939

PERMABOOK edition published September, 1948
16th printing........................July, 1960

L

PERMABOOK editions are distributed in the U.S. by Affiliated Publishers, Inc., 630 Fifth Avenue, New York 20, N.Y.

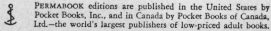

PERMABOOK editions are published in the United States by Pocket Books, Inc., and in Canada by Pocket Books of Canada, Ltd.—the world's largest publishers of low-priced adult books.

TO MY FATHER AND THOSE PIONEERS, DOCTORS OR OTHERWISE, WHO BRAVED THE RIDICULE OF THEIR CONTEMPORARIES TO HEAL THE AILING WITH DIET, AND THUS BLAZED THE WAY FOR THE SCIENCE OF NUTRITION.

Contents

vii

Preface

TO BEFUDDLE FATTIES with reducing diets which cannot possibly work, in order to further the sales of fattening foods, has become a major occupation. It is a form of cheating that may injure people who should lose weight.

Some people vow that no diet can help them. Bosh! The right kind of reducing diet cannot fail. But only a real understanding of foods and body fat can insure your being able to distinguish the right from the wrong kind. You had better find out the facts, for, to use the vernacular, we fatties are being played for suckers—and big ones, at that!

You may think that I hold the unusual body chemical processes of the overweight person in low esteem. Not at all! On the contrary, I consider fat men and women as specially gifted people—super-super metabolic enigmas. They are able to transform food into fat (which is stored energy) at a much more efficient rate than the thin or normal individual. With this exceptional talent, they might even live longer and fare better than non-overweights—*provided they hold their weight to normal.*

The trouble is that fat people allow their unique ability to make them fat. And an ability that always has to be watched becomes a nuisance. So let us agree with the common verdict that the tendency to take on fat is a fault.

The Food Calorie Is a Giant

—Not a little pest, as many discussers of diet seem to believe. A recent book on reducing by a well-known medical man defines a "calorie" as "the amount of heat required to raise one gram of water 1 degree Centigrade." From the author's later conclusions and comparisons, it is evident that he meant this definition to hold for a food calorie.

What he was really describing is the *physical* calorie, which is technically known as the gram-calorie.

A *food* calorie is the amount of heat required to raise 1000 grams of water 1 degree Centigrade—just 1000 times as big as most writers on reducing seem to consider it.

Inside the living human body, where a constant temperature of at least 98.6 degrees Fahrenheit is maintained, body fat is an oily liquid. True, it is held in place by delicate adipose tissue, which might be likened to the wax cubicles of a honeycomb, but body fat itself is liquid.

This fundamental fact makes a difference—as you will presently read.

V. H. L.

EAT—AND REDUCE!

CHAPTER ONE

Misery Has Company

DEAR READER: What is written here is passed on to you by a fellow who is in the same boat with you, O fat one! If at times I seem a bit harsh, or, to use slang, rather tough, on the obese, please remember that there is a certain degree of self-castigation involved.

With the same problem you have and a huge curiosity about why things are as they are, I had compelling personal reasons for being interested in *fat*. Being born, so to speak, into a profession where it was necessary to know something about foods and reducing, was a further stimulation to study fat. And finally, through the medium of radio broadcasting, came the most magnificent opportunity anyone ever had to study fat people. That is the why of this book.

We fat people are in a class by ourselves. Those lucky mortals who have no worries about taking on weight will never, never know what they have escaped. They who can sit down to three meals a day and eat pretty nearly what they please, with no concern over weight, have their nutrition problems, too, but they are probably not aware of any. At least that pest of nutrition, the calorie, does not bother them.

We fat people are a large class, both in substance and in numbers. If we estimate the population of the United States at the rough figure of 130 million, we can say that 80 million are over the age of 21. We will never know exactly because the birth rate is going down while more children are being kept alive, which together with the fact that the average span of life is being increased, does strange things to our life tables. It affects obesity statistics, also, for middle age brings fat to many people.

Very soon one third of the people in the United States will be over the age of 50, which brings its share of problems. These shifting balances make it difficult to approximate the number of fat people despite the voluminous data insurance statistics give us. The best we can do is make some pretty good guesses.

If we accept the estimate of 80 million adults, we can figure quite accurately that approximately 16 million are overweight and 37 million are underweight. The figure of 37 million underweight is surprising, but it is essentially correct.

The defect of being underweight does not receive the attention that obesity does. Most insurance companies divide overweight people into three classes: (1)

those from 5 to 14 per cent overweight; (2) those from 15 to 24 per cent overweight; and (3) those 25 per cent and more overweight.

The insurance doctor has a complicated but very efficient way of estimating the individual percentage of overweight. He does not draw his conclusions by consulting simple age-height-weight tables such as those on the penny weight scales. He determines the degree of overweight by comparing body weight with the height, the width of the shoulders, and the distance between the tips of the hip bones. If you really want to know how much overweight you are, consult a doctor who understands this method of computing weight normals. You may, if you wish, get an approximate idea of how you stand from the weight charts near the end of this book.

If you should fall into class 1, class 2, or class 3, as the case may be, it is very significant as far as your chances for long life and health are concerned. The more overweight you are, the greater the hazard to your health and life.

Out of the 16 million overweight adults, close to 11 million will fall into class 1. Their death rate is 22 per cent higher than that of normal people. About 4 million fall into class 2, with a death rate increase of 44 per cent. Somewhat over a million fat people are in class 3. Their death rate jumps 74 per cent. About one

3

person out of a hundred fat people is 50 per cent or more overweight.

In addition, from 6 to 7 million overfat babies, youngsters, and youths may be added to the list of obese adults. These make an impressive total.

For those who are trying to reduce, we really have something—not only a first-class reducing diet but far more than that: a plan which will enable *you* to wage war easily, successfully, and comfortably on fat.

The fat person who sets forth every once in a while grimly resolved to starve and deny himself, and winds up after the punishment with ten pounds gone, is not uncommon. Perhaps a month later the prodigal pounds have returned. Fatty pouts "Oh, what's the use" for a little while. Then, suddenly, when an extra chin bulges forth or the belt has to be let out another inch, he sadly, desperately, takes another fling at his reducing scheme—or a new one.

So life goes for him. Two steps forward, three steps backward. Eventually, he winds up behind the 228-pound ball. That sort of existence need no longer be your lot.

I promise further that you may, if you wish, go through life henceforth with the same attitude that I personally have toward controlling fat—a gay, happy, confident one. Fat really is just a miserable form of SUET, essentially weak and cowardly liquid, that

4

clutters up your body. It is readily destroyed and prevented.

Some forms of body fat are a little tougher than others but the hardiest can be turned into water, some carbonic acids, and gases very easily by putting certain body chemical processes in motion.

About sixty years ago a brilliant scientist, Carl Voit of Munich, demonstrated that geese, who ate corn and grain, could make the starch in the grains into goose fat. Right then and there science started on the road to understanding the problems of overweight. Animal food chemistry was found to parallel that of human beings.

Other chemists studied the chemistry of the sugars in fruits and other foods. In fact, contributions from most of the great chemists of the last century brought light to our understanding of fat—light that told us beyond contradiction that the problem of body fat is one of food chemistry and that alone.

Yes, basically the problem of body fat is one of food and eating habits. No matter how much we worm and squirm and try to evade the issue, that fact remains.

Since men have existed, there have been fat ones and thin ones. The earliest of Egyptian drawings depict an occasional fat figure. The Talmud tells of a rabbi so obese that his "belly was opened and baskets of fat were removed." The Bible tells of Israel, who ate

5

fats and sweets until he grew waxy pale and so enormously fat that he was "disgusting before the Lord."

Always a few have suspected the connection between food and body fat. But mostly the relation has been denied. Very likely King Tut's fat aunt maintained that she "ate like a bird." Our ancestors may be forgiven, for they were handicapped in understanding fat. Hippocrates, the father of medicine, had taught that there was only one kind of body nourishment, a "universal ailment" extracted from any and all foods, and that this primary substance nourished the body.

Scientists believed this theory until about a hundred years ago. Then they slowly began to change their minds. Along about 1800, a scientist, Einhoff, fed a cow different grasses and grains for stated periods of time. He demonstrated that foods had different values, although for quite a few years this monumental knowledge was used only in animal husbandry.

Strange as it may seem, the *first* reducing diet that received any medical or scientific notice appeared in 1863 (the Banting diet). How slow is the march of knowledge! Even more strange is the fact that the principles of this first recognized reducing diet, crude and inefficient, still exercise authority.

Dr. William Banting, enormously fat, reduced himself by cutting down on starches and fats. He lived practically on meat alone. He took off pounds all right

—but he eventually killed himself with his unbalanced diet. Nevertheless, Banting became the authority on reducing; we can thank him for a start in the right direction and thank our stars that modern nutrition has guided us into safer channels.

To give you a sort of preview of what is coming, let me say that our way of controlling weight is based on an understanding of the behavior of various foods in the body. Certain fruits and vegetables stir a series of reactions in the body which literally burn fat. It is true that we use the calorie as a measuring rule—but that is as far as it goes. Our way is really an *Eat* and Reduce method. You can carry on in the spirit of a knight who is out to joust with the ogre Obesity. To me, fighting fat is a game of wits, an adventure of which I never tire.

I can add up the score every night by standing on the scales. If I have held my own in weight that day, I am content. If I have taken off a pound, hurrah! Taken on a pound? So what? At least I know why I did, and it's easy to dissolve that extra tallow, with foods. It is interesting to let Old Man Fat gain a point, too, once in a while, especially if he wins via a delectable piece of pie à la mode. No, it is not exactly painful to take a setback—once in a while. The manipulation of body chemistry by eating certain foods is intensely fascinating.

7

On our side are the thinning foods; on Old Man Fat's, the fattening ones. Numerically, the opponents have an advantage, but that is a challenge. Strategy and good generalship win here, as in any competition.

In the United States, we have, more or less readily available, about 250 foods to tempt us, nourish us, and give us our health. Various combinations of these foods, of course, and ingenious ways of preparing them, run the number of edible dishes up into thousands. Fundamentally, there are about 100 common body-fat destroying foods. Perhaps fifty foods that we should eat to balance our diets are "neutral." The rest are worthy opponents. If we fall for the opponents' blandishments, we grow fat. To be slim, we have to stick to our partners, and dodge the fattening troublemakers. Knowing right well who is who among foods, we just stalk our way among the opponents and deftly elude them. We can dine at the Stork Club or its like and take the menu in stride. It comes of knowing foods —that's all.

You can chose an hors d'oeuvre, a soup, entrée, salad, and dessert that cannot put weight on you. Dinner at a good eating place is an extra challenge. It tests your mettle and skill. Incidentally, head waiters, their assistants, and the others who flutter around you with suggestions and temptations respect the person who is choosy about his food. You can win their coöperation by saying, "I am watching my diet, but I am in the mood for a good meal. Let's see what you can do."

The trouble with most people who are trying to stay normal in weight is that they don't know enough about foods to distinguish friend from foe. They are quite lost when confronted with a menu or with the task of buying a day's food at the grocery.

It is a pretty glum life for them, too, because they are defeated before they start. To them, it seems all the foods in the world, except perhaps six, are fattening. The austere, gloomy, thinning foods they do know are probably abominable. Dieting when you don't know your foods is like playing cards when you don't know an ace from a jack.

Many a person not burdened with a tendency to fat can't conceive of anyone going through life defending himself against foods. But we fatties know what it means. Can you go about your eating with the happy frame of mind and confidence I have? Do you believe it is possible?

It is. I am telling you no lies! Promise to read this book carefully, to give it some study—and I promise that, henceforth, you can enjoy eating and still control fat! Thousands of people are doing so. Their progress is a matter of record.

9

Perhaps the campaign we have worked out to stay within reasonable bounds of weight may not appeal to you, as far as individual food tastes are concerned. That doesn't matter, really. The principles involved are what is important. You will easily learn the rules —then play your own way. Use the foods you like; the choice is wide.

How the program works out practically, I can best tell you from my personal experiences. At the moment of writing, I weigh 176 pounds stripped.

Seven years ago, my weight hovered around 190 pounds. I felt good so gave no thought to trimming down. Then in 1932 I took a long vacation. A friend took a snapshot of me in a bathing suit as I loafed in a beach chair one July day. He was cruel enough to give me a print of the picture. Ugh! I had that most embarrassing of all experiences—seeing my obesity as others see it. Privately I sought a scale. I weighed 207 pounds. I, who knew that it isn't healthy to be fat, was ashamed. It was time for me to reduce. I did.

I have used the Lindlahr seven-day reducing diet three times to take off no less than seven or eight pounds in seven days. Since 1932 I have used the principles involved to watch my dietetic P's and Q's and have easily and pleasantly maintained the weight I desired. Best of all, I have always enjoyed each day's eating to the full, for I believe implicitly that good eating is one of the few joys in which mankind should revel, within limits.

Most people who "take on weight" do so after they pass the age of 30. At some time in the twenties the body tissues stop growing and developing. We usually become less active, too. By then, an individual is definitely past the age when he needs a surplus of nourishment.

Growing youngsters should, of course, eat more than their bodies require for energy and replacement alone. They are *developing*. Unfortunately, the habits of eating acquired in youth stick to us, and we may continue to eat extra food as adults. In many of us, such surplus becomes fat.

We fatties have a basic problem—how do we get that way? We have to look at many factors to find out the answer. Therefore, in addition to presenting diet facts, it is going to be necessary to speculate a bit on why people grow fat, for somewhere among the reasons why fat people in general are fat is the reason or reasons why you and I in particular are fat. Or, if you please, why we have that vexing *tendency* to grow fat.

The phrase "tendency to fat" is one that strikes at the very roots of the problem. However, it is clumsy to write; so, for the sake of convenience, let's coin a word that fits the thought.

"Lipos" is the Greek word for fat, and most chemical

terms relating to fat are built around it. The word "lipophil" is defined in the dictionary as "having an affinity for fat, absorbing fat." By adding the suffix "ic," we have a word, *lipophilic* (pronounced lip-o-fill'-ik, with "lip" as in "tulip"), which we will henceforth use either as an adjective or noun, as is done with the word "alcoholic." That's us, O fat ones—we are lipophilic. I am lipophilic. If you have a tendency to take on weight too readily, you also are lipophilic. Remember the word, because that's what we are—lipophilics.

While on the subject of words, let me explain the term "Debble Fat." I may use it often; it's an ingrained habit with me now.

Debble Fat is a name that was coined by Lorna Doone J. . . ., a perfect prototype of Aunt Jemima, and a cook in my household for many delightful years. I never did find out her weight (she wouldn't even bother to determine it), but it must have been well in excess of 300 pounds.

How Lorna could cook—ah, sweet memories! She liked to be fat and she liked to eat fattening foods. Thinning foods earned her special scorn. She'd pout out her lips when making a salad, and mutter "Rabbit food." She would "lip" even farther when cooking spinach, cabbage, or greens. "Horse food" was her bitter comment.

Left unguarded, Lorna would wield the grease ladle, the butter spoon, and the olive oil can as a reaper wields his scythe. But we deterred her, almost forcibly. She would regretfully pass by the butter, the lard, and the bacon drippings which she tenderly saved. Not without remonstrance, though—she would point sadly to the grease pots and say, "Debble Fat's doings, but it's good."

Lorna would countenance no interference with her own private eating. That was her business. And she had grown so content with her excess fat that it would have been cruel to interfere.

Besides, she had an unsurpassed gift for choosing the most fattening of foods. Catch her in the kitchen at four o'clock in the afternoon, with a good thick slice of bread laden with butter and goose liver, and Lorna would roll ecstatic eyes: "Debble Fat's doings. But it's good."

To her, the god of fat was no sinister monster; he was just a gay tempter whose ultimate objective she couldn't fathom. And she didn't care. Debble Fat's doings were delightful.

CHAPTER TWO

"Debble Fat" Has Allies

THE CARDS are stacked against us fatties. If ever the
path of a pilgrim was made discouragingly hard, surely
it is the straight and narrow road to slimness. Against
us, it seems, society is arrayed—custom, convenience,
habits and trends, even "business."

Tens of millions of dollars are spent during each
year to make us fatties eat what we shouldn't, and, I
vow, it is a shortsighted policy. Those officials of trade
associations and "food institutes," manufacturers and
salesmen who stay awake nights devising campaigns,
and set aside heavy budgets to entice fat people to eat
their products, would be better off to let us alone.

Fat people die too young, and if our 16 million fat
people have shortened their life spans by only five
years each, that cuts off big and small business of every
sort from a tremendous potential income. Let us figure
for a minute. Sixteen million times five years equals
80 million human life years.

Three meals a day would be eaten by each person
during the 365 days of each one of those 80 million

human life years. Rent would be paid, clothes bought, money spent, and the sum involved would run into such staggering totals that an Einstein would be needed to calculate them. And mind you, we are very conservative in allocating only five extra years of life to the average fat person who reduces.

The figures are as follows: For each pound of over-weight after the age of 35, life expectancy is decreased by 1 per cent. To illustrate, a woman of 35 whose normal weight is 134 pounds has a normal life expectancy of twenty-eight years. If she allows her weight to increase to 184 pounds, that is, fifty pounds more than her optimum weight, her life expectancy is reduced to approximately fourteen years. This is not theory; this comes from exact insurance statistics, which are almost in a class of sureties with death and taxes. Striving to tempt the fat person to stay fat is poor business.

Those groups which buy the services of well-known scientists, great universities, or respected medical journals to "prove" that bread, cookies, macaroni, cereals, and so on, are not fattening, are not only straining the truth to the breaking point but are also deluding themselves.

Lipophilics who live longer, even those who watch their calories, are going to eat more of the fattening foods during their extra years of life than they will in

15

the Great Beyond. Even the fat person devotedly concerned with reducing will relax his vigilance once in a while, cheat a little bit and indulge in those foods it would be wiser for him not to eat.

Finally, the reducer will, sooner or later, reach a satisfactory weight. At that time, he can and should eat more of the fattening foods. These are logical and simple truths, but there is no hope, I am sure, of convincing august boards of directors who shudder in a heart-rending fashion every time the fact is mentioned that their product is fattening.

Besides, most fat people are not so credulous as they are presumed to be. They sniff a rodent when they are told that the proper reducing diet should include three pieces of bread per meal. Even though a most respected university is the sponsor of, let's say, the baloney-and-eggs reducing diet, John Fat Public is apt to suspect that this is a not too subtle way of convincing the unwary that baloney isn't fattening.

Here, approximately, is the way certain "diets" are born. Genial, go-getting I. Sellum, sales manager of the Consolidated Baloney Corporation, announces at the annual directors' meeting:

Gentlemen, I am sorry to report that the impression is still strong in the public mind that baloney is fattening! There's no question that a great many people in the United States are attempting in some way or another to

16

avoid what they consider fattening foods. You know, as well as I do, that baloney, with its high energy fat, is one of the most nutritious foods in the world. Clearly Nature intended, among other things, that no eggs should be served without baloney.

Yet, good sirs, observers placed by us in strategic locations at various restaurants reported that only one person in ten ordered baloney with his eggs. Gentlemen, fried eggs ungraced by baloney are definitely a distinct menace to the bread and butter of 32,000 employees in this great industry of ours. Furthermore, the widows and orphans who hold the majority of our stock are literally robbed when naked fried eggs are served to the consuming public.

Fellow workers, our deadliest enemy is that entity—nebulous and difficult to describe, but a force withal—the reducing craze!

We can pull the fangs of this viper in our bosom. We can destroy it. Sitting beside me is the eminent scientist, Professor Pushover Fordough. I have discussed at length with him the nutritional chemistry of baloney, and he has assured me that when eggs and baloney are eaten together, the fat in the baloney is literally exploded!

Gentlemen, for the fat person, baloney and eggs are an ideal reducing dish. I am going to ask your permission now to engage the services of Professor Fordough. I can guarantee that stupendous publicity will be given to his important research—and good sirs, I repeat, millions of fat people are at this moment neglecting to order baloney with their eggs (because of the hysterical propaganda of food faddists).

By our plan, within three months we will have shown these poor misguided mortals the error of their ways. And

17

if only one out of three eats one extra piece of baloney henceforth, those pieces laid end to end would reach from New York to Los Angeles and half way back to Kansas City.

Gentlemen, your pleasure!

Well, good reader, that sort of baloney is the least of our troubles, popular as it is. Machinations not so deliberate, or just unpremeditated and natural difficulties, make it toughest for us. After all, for every one of us who has to watch his diet, there are four who don't. Restaurants cannot gear their menus and reform their styles of cooking to cater to us fatties. It wouldn't be good business!

So they give us short shrift, and we can't blame them. If the great mass of restaurant patrons want fattening foods, rich desserts, heavy gravies, and cooking done with a liberal use of fats, oils, and butter, what chance do we, a small minority, stand? Not much!

Mrs. Ima Hostess has the same problem. Two of her dinner guests are fatties; two are not. Since her family is decidedly "not," she's going to run into trouble if she even considers planning a reducing menu. No, the majority rules—sometimes even without a copy of Roberts' Rules of Order.

Yes, it seems as if menus, dinners, parties, picnics, and all arrangements for group eating were planned with an eye to the person who is not lipophilic. Yet we can't eat alone. Half the charm of any meal is sharing the enjoyment of eating with friends.

When Lord Bolingbroke once wanted to tempt Dean Swift to dinner, he showed him, as an inducement, an elaborate bill of fare. Dean Swift replied, "A fig for your bill of fare; show me your bill of company." Right!

Not only social forces oppose us, but so does Father Time. The young are able to eat much more food without gaining weight than those of us who are older. Obviously, they are growing and some of their food is used in development. They are also more active by virtue of the inclinations and the opportunities of youth.

But most important of all, their metabolism rate is higher. That is vitally important to remember. You're going to have to understand this term, *metabolism rate,* if you are really going to comprehend the phenomenon of fat. So why not do it now?

First, let us define metabolism. Metabolism is the term used to include in one word all the multitudinous chemical processes within the body which determine the growth and replacement of body tissues, the production of body heat and energy necessary for muscular activity and all other vital functions.

19

In a sense, then, what lay people call the life processes of the body, scientists call the metabolism. Obviously, one person's metabolism may be more active or less active than another's. The metabolism, then, has a *rate*. The rate may be average, slow or fast, as the case may be. Just as you might judge how much steam is up in a steam boat by the amount of smoke coming from the smoke funnel, so scientists have a way of determining the human metabolism rate.

The amount of carbon dioxide thrown off in the breath keeps pace with the heat production in the body. An apparatus has been devised to measure faithfully this output. Consequently, by considering a person's height and approximate skin area in relation to his carbon dioxide output, his internal heat production can be determined. This accurately determines his personal metabolism rate.

The rate of metabolism in the body when a person is at absolute physical and mental rest is called the *basal* metabolism rate. The basal metabolism rate should be determined in reality when a person is in deep, sound, restful sleep. However, it cannot easily be measured then, so when you go to your doctor to have a basal metabolism test, it is made while you are resting, although awake.

A metabolism test is usually made twelve hours after you have eaten a light meal and in a room at about 70 degrees F. It will then be about 10 per cent higher than when you are in restful sleep.

However, whatever it is at the time of a proper test is called your basal metabolism rate. Doctors use a symbol to express it, the letters B.M.R. A person's B.M.R. gives some important diagnostic clues to the doctor.

All in all, roughly, the heat production of the average adult is one calorie per hour for every two and two-tenths pounds of body weight. In a metabolism test, a man weighing 110 pounds, who produces about fifty calories of body heat per hour, is considered average. His metabolism rate is called normal.

Another man of the same height and weight who produces fifty-five calories of body heat per hour is considered to have a high metabolism (10 per cent plus). Still another man who produces only about forty-five calories of body heat per hour has what is called a slow or minus metabolism (10 per cent minus).

Think of a fire for a moment. Chemically, burning is a violent form of combustion. A very gentle form of combustion is *oxidation*. It is by oxidation that body heat is produced—that warmth of life, the 98.6 degrees temperature your body has in health.

You know how a fire burns brightly and quickly in a draft. In a sense, the basal metabolism rate is the draft in which body fires burn (oxidation takes place). Just as fireplaces have drafts which vary in effectiveness, so we human beings have distinctive basal metabolisms, some quite efficient, some not so good.

The rate of your basal metabolism has much to do with the question of food and body fat accumulation. Basically, body fat is food which has not been turned into heat or energy.

One of the greatest chemists of all time, Antoine Laurent Lavoisier, was the genius who gave us our first understanding of the fact that food produces heat in the body. If Parisian revolutionists had not cut off his head one November day in 1792, science might have been saved a hundred years of slow plodding. But even though Lavoisier was guillotined, we will remember at least one of his many scientific discoveries —that body heat is produced from the foods we eat.

Now if food is the fuel source of human body heat, and metabolism the medium that converts food into heat, there must be a definite relation between the basal metabolism rate and fat production—and there is, a decided one.

A normal metabolism rate helps you greatly to stay just about normal in weight. A slow metabolism rate makes you tend to put on pounds, and a high metabolism rate is apt to keep you thin.

Students of obesity are puzzled by the fact that fat

people often have normal or plus basal metabolism rates. To my mind, this is not strange because the basal metabolism rate is a comparatively crude measurement of the *total* metabolism. A component of the total, such as the fat metabolism, may be functioning abnormally without affecting the complete picture, just as the perverted sugar metabolism in diabetes is not reflected in the basal metabolism rate.

On the average, females have a lower metabolic rate than males of the same age. Orientals and Negroes have a lower metabolism rate, which helps to explain why they may grow fatter, when they do grow fat, than white people. Athletes and hard-working people usually have a higher basal metabolism rate than people who lead a more sedentary life.

But however high our B.M.R. may be when begin life, it grows less and less as life goes on. In infancy it is higher than in adolescence, and in adulthood lower than in youth. At every decade in life the B.M.R. is less, and as far as we are concerned this means that the tendency to accumulate fat will be increased.

So the older we get, the more difficulty we have in holding down poundage. The forties make lipophilics out of many people. That is why we admit Father Time, too, is against us.

These are just a few of the hazards we are up

against. No wonder odds are heavy that we will stay fat!

It all sounds pretty gloomy, but take heart. We have had some good breaks, too. Let's look further.

"Debble Fat" Takes a Setback

THIRTY YEARS AGO it was all right to be fat. Today, it is not. Although many lipophilics allow the...elves to get fat today, the percentage was higher in the 1.. ..'s. It took an aroused group of stout womenfolk to lead a large contingent of amazingly overfat Americans toward a saner and safer national average weight. For that, God bless the ladies. Some of the lean Uncle Sam's of tradition had gradually waxed fatter and fatter until they looked more like the proverbial John Bull. Certain Mrs. Uncle Sam's had fared no better. They had been placed on a pedestal and overfed.

Perhaps it was because we had conquered raw country, and hardy pioneers had become complacent merchants, lawyers, doctors, and bankers. Perhaps we remembered the English tradition that obesity spelled prosperity.

Those were the days of good eating. Diamond Jim Brady was a national hero, and "double portions of plenty" were the vogue. Here is an August day's menu taken from a cook book printed in 1905:

25

BREAKFAST
peaches and cream
boiled grits   *fried eggs*
broiled mutton chop   *fried potatoes*
biscuits

LIGHT LUNCHEON
small assorted sandwiches
corned beef and cabbage   *boiled potatoes*
bread pudding

DINNER
radishes   *salted peanuts*
bean soup
filet of halibut   *potato croquettes*
breast of lamb
chicken livers sauté
green corn in cream   *green peas*
watercress salad
tapioca pudding

What food for August! Imagine my father, with his almost newly painted shingle "H. Lindlahr, M.D." hanging outside the door at 232 South Michigan Avenue in Chicago, setting forth to tell overstout "nice people" of that city to eat spinach, salads, and greens.

I remember a fat Caruso of that day singing romantic parts, a hefty Isadora Duncan doing esthetic dancing. It seems to me Teddy Roosevelt was no lightweight, and his cabinet—from William Howard Taft down— did justice to the national standard of well-being.

26

Significant of the times were the chorus girls. They were hefty to say the least, and Billy Watson's Beef Trust was an aggregation of girls who averaged at least 200 pounds each, or was it more? Buxomness was the "it" of the day.

The vice of overweight was not limited to adults alone. If you care to take the trouble of looking up the class picture of Vassar '04, '05, or 'o anything, you'll get a rough idea of the situation. Even about-to-be-born babies were fat. The ladies in my mother's circle used to look with scorn upon any mother whose baby weighed less than ten pounds at birth. One obscure lady in our neighborhood produced a sixteen-pound baby, and she rose swiftly to be Madame President of the Tuesday Sewing Circle.

My mother was always rather slim. One year, perhaps it was 1906, she blossomed forth in a *directoire* gown, but the lifted eyebrows of her amply-cushioned friends soon discouraged her. As a rule, if I remember rightly, Mother was quite busy with bustles, mysterious furbelows, ruffles and puffed sleeves, ingeniously trying to look fatter than she was. Stylemakers tried, sporadically, to cast a pall of shame upon obesity, but were not too successful.

Then, all of a sudden, things began to happen. It would take a better historian than I to record, and assess the relative importance of, the steps that led to a tremendous change in the national attitude toward fat. Dozens of factors entered into it.

Fashion experts were raising their voices in earnest. Women began to bob their hair—they found short hair made them look much younger. They began to realize, too, that slimness lent the appearance of youth.

The World War of 1914 sent fat a-scurrying. After all, girls were replacing men in industry, were driving ambulances in France. Fat women couldn't squeeze into the pert uniforms of the day or appear engaging (or efficient) in the office force or factory set-up.

Even greater forces were at work. Women were striving for equal recognition with men, not alone in the vote, but in the right to work and play at the side of the stronger sex. They were bound and determined to enjoy sports and other such privileges, including perhaps the double standard, that men had long held sacred to themselves. Perhaps throwing off the burden of immense wads of hair, and corresponding wads of fat, was a further expression of freedom and the New Deal for womankind.

Yes, in those fateful years, an impressive number of women were certainly coming out of the kitchen and the home. They were no longer content to sit in the parlor and grow fat.

Once a few of the sisterhood had grown slim, trim, and attractive from these measures, all enterprising mendous change in the national attitude toward fat. Dozens of factors entered into it.

Fashion experts were raising their voices in earnest. Women began to bob their hair—they found short hair made them look much younger. They began to realize, too, that slimness lent the appearance of youth.

The World War of 1914 sent fat a-scurrying. After all, girls were replacing men in industry, were driving ambulances in France. Fat women couldn't squeeze into the pert uniforms of the day or appear engaging (or efficient) in the office force or factory set-up.

Even greater forces were at work. Women were striving for equal recognition with men, not alone in the vote, but in the right to work and play at the side of the stronger sex. They were bound and determined to enjoy sports and other such privileges, including perhaps the double standard, that men had long held sacred to themselves. Perhaps throwing off the burden of immense wads of hair, and corresponding wads of fat, was a further expression of freedom and the New Deal for womankind.

Yes, in those fateful years, an impressive number of women were certainly coming out of the kitchen and the home. They were no longer content to sit in the parlor and grow fat.

Once a few of the sisterhood had grown slim, trim, and attractive from these measures, all enterprising

Significant of the times were the chorus girls. They were hefty to say the least, and Billy Watson's Beef Trust was an aggregation of girls who averaged at least 200 pounds each, or was it more? Buxomness was the "it" of the day.

The vice of overweight was not limited to adults alone. If you care to take the trouble of looking up the class picture of Vassar '01, '05, or 'o anything, you'll get a rough idea of the situation. Even about-to-be-born babies were fat. The ladies in my mother's circle used to look with scorn upon any mother whose baby weighed less than ten pounds at birth. One obscure lady in our neighborhood produced a sixteen-pound baby, and she rose swiftly to be Madame President of the Tuesday Sewing Circle.

My mother was always rather slim. One year, perhaps it was 1906, she blossomed forth in a *directoire* gown, but the lifted eyebrows of her amply-cushioned friends soon discouraged her. As a rule, if I remember rightly, Mother was quite busy with bustles, mysterious furbelows, ruffles and puffed sleeves, ingeniously trying to look fatter than she was. Stylemakers tried, sporadically, to cast a pall of shame upon obesity, but were not too successful.

Then, all of a sudden, things began to happen. It would take a better historian than I to record, and assess the relative importance of, the steps that led to a tre-

27

BREAKFAST
peaches and cream
boiled grits   *fried eggs*
broiled mutton chop   *fried potatoes*
biscuits

LIGHT LUNCHEON
small assorted sandwiches
corned beef and cabbage   *boiled potatoes*
bread pudding

DINNER
radishes   *salted peanuts*
bean soup
filet of halibut   *potato croquettes*
breast of lamb
chicken livers sauté
green corn in cream   *green peas*
watercress salad
tapioca pudding

What food for August! Imagine my father, with his almost newly painted shingle "H. Lindlahr, M.D." hanging outside the door at 232 South Michigan Avenue in Chicago, setting forth to tell overstout "nice people" of that city to eat spinach, salads, and greens.

I remember a fat Caruso of that day singing romantic parts, a hefty Isadora Duncan doing esthetic dancing. It seems to me Teddy Roosevelt was no lightweight, and his cabinet—from William Howard Taft down—did justice to the national standard of well-being.

"Debble Fat" Takes a Setback

THIRTY YEARS AGO it was all right to be fat. Today, it is not. Although many lipophilics allow themselves to get fat today, the percentage was higher in the 1900's. It took an aroused group of stout womenfolk to lead a large contingent of amazingly overfat Americans toward a saner and safer national average weight. For that, God bless the ladies. Some of the lean Uncle Sam's of tradition had gradually waxed fatter and fatter until they looked more like the proverbial John Bull. Certain Mrs. Uncle Sam's had fared no better. They had been placed on a pedestal and overfed.

Perhaps it was because we had conquered raw country, and hardy pioneers had become complacent merchants, lawyers, doctors, and bankers. Perhaps we remembered the English tradition that obesity spelled prosperity.

Those were the days of good eating. Diamond Jim Brady was a national hero, and "double portions of plenty" were the vogue. Here is an August day's menu taken from a cook book printed in 1905:

women promptly followed suit, pell mell. Irene Castle, with her slimness and her saucily-bobbed hair, epitomized the trend. Even the new dances she introduced seemed to further the doom of portliness.

The stately waltz lost out to more agile dances such as the Castle Walk and the tango. Couples began to dance in restaurants, and women who wanted to indulge in that pleasure had to train and trim down their girth. And so, a host of factors led to an unceasing, grim, devouring urge to slimness which gathered momentum until it was grossly exaggerated. Yes, the tide went too far.

With a later generation of young women (the astonishing flappers) seeking to abolish natural contours and trying, desperately, to emulate the shape of a fence rail, the situation was bad. Perhaps Mae West helped to turn the psychological tide. At least her advent proved a long-sought delight to the eyes of millions of men who had longed for the sight of a movie star with curves.

I am told on good authority that many men, a bit older than I, were muttering in their sleep in the 1920's, "Lillian Russell, where art thou?"

Today we seem headed for a better, more sensible national feminine figure, one that is just about right.

But we were discussing the first wholesome reaction against Victorian obesity. Although it would be interesting to know exactly how it all came about, the guesses we have advanced are probably as good as any. The point is, a national urge to slimness finally came.

From the beginning, this splendid reform has been most unjustly attacked, and libelously termed "the craze" for reducing. How I despise that phrase! It's debasing to a worthy endeavor, insulting to the laudatory aspirations of good, sensible people.

"Craze" is a nasty word. It smacks of irrationality, foolishness, imbecility and whatnot. The urge to reduce, which overtook a fat American citizenry some twenty years ago, was one of the healthiest changes that ever happened to our nation. Whatever brought it about—whether the factors were trivial and frivolous or deep-seated biological urges of self-preservation (as I'm inclined to believe they were)—whatever the factors were, they were for the best.

I shudder to think what would have happened to us modern lipophilics if we had been as complacent about fat as our parents of the mauve decade were. We probably would have averaged more than 200 pounds apiece on the hoof if what did happen to change our minds hadn't happened.

For within the last thirty years, events, inventions and the general progress of civilization have conspired to help make the royal road to obesity almost impossible to escape for those with a tendency for fat. The butcher, the baker, the candy and ice cream maker tempt us as never before. Transportation, refrigeration, and the arts and wiles of merchandising, including that of advertising, almost catapult alluring—and fattening —tidbits into our mouths.

Automobiles, machines, household gadgets are doing their best to abolish the need for physical activity, which would burn up some fat. Shorter hours of work, more granted or enforced leisure, do not help to keep us thin. Factors which lead to fatness have been on the increase; they are not apt to become fewer.

Today, Americans eat three times as much fatty food per person over a twelve-month period as they did fifty years ago. Today, Americans eat eight times as much sugar per person per year as they did 100 years ago. We are ripe for a movement to resist the trend.

So let's drink a hearty toast to the "urge" for reducing. Let's celebrate its birth and its continued existence, and wish it an everlasting life! Providence must have planned it. . . .

Well, we've covered some important generalities. You must suspect by now that to fight fat intelligently it is necessary to consider the problem of obesity as a whole.

Defeating "Debble Fat" isn't alone a matter of dieting. Social and environmental factors also have to be considered. In fact, psychological problems are just about as important as the dietetic ones. The adage "Man's worst enemy is himself" holds as true in the war against fat as in other avenues of life. Yes, the mind, the character, and the personal equation of the fat person just have to be reckoned with, and sometimes adjusted.

We are going to have to look very closely at some fat individuals to learn a few lessons. But first we can settle back for a comforting little interlude of looking at those lipophilics over there.

Let me tell you a little story. . . .

CHAPTER FOUR

The Liverwurst Ladies

ONE DAY, in the early spring of 1935, I had lunch at the soda fountain counter of a department store near my office. There was an empty stool at my left and two vacant ones at my right.

I was contenting myself with a delicious salad when in swooped three ladies. "Swooped" is the word, for they must have totalled at least 675 pounds of concentrated womanhood. Two of them squeezed into place on the stools at the right. The third one started to maneuver herself into the space at my left.

Since they all overflowed the accommodations considerably, a bit of discretion was obviously in order—I stepped back from my stool and offered it to the lady at my left. She accepted most graciously, and then the fun began. Of course I listened. Soda fountains are not exactly ivory towers of isolation.

Said the first lady to the soda clerk, "I'll have a liverwurst sandwich with pickle relish on white bread with no lettuce and *no butter,* a large glass of soda with ice in it, please. And don't forget, *no butter!*"

Said the second hefty one, "Well, that sounds like a good idea. Waiter, I'll have the same."

They looked expectantly at their friend, who was studying the menu with visible perturbation. Finally, No. 3 looked up appealingly and said, "I'd just love to have that creamed shrimp, but I never eat shrimp away from home. You're having liverwurst? Waiter, I'll have the same, with relish and mayonnaise—no butter."

While they were waiting for the orders to come, they busied themselves with a discussion about Sarah. Sarah, I gathered, had accompanied them to the knitting class upstairs, but couldn't join them for lunch because her knees were hurting badly. She was going to rest a little bit and then go home.

The first Liverwurst Lady carried most of the conversational burden. "So sorry for Sarah. . . . Her rheumatism really is bad. . . . Really, though, Sarah ought to reduce. . . . She must have gained 100 pounds since she moved to Brooklyn. She used to have the loveliest figure." . . . And so on.

The liverwurst-and-mayonnaise lady broke in. She just knew Sarah would die of a broken heart. Sam left her alone all the time. He always had some excuse to be out and away from home—conferences, conventions, business. He never took her any place.

Then they all chirped up and put Sarah's husband on the pan. Just as the waiter hove in sight with the liverwurst sandwiches, the first queen of the liver-wursts concluded mournfully that Sam was such a nice little fellow when he and Sarah first moved to Brooklyn.

By that time, the sandwiches were before them, the ladies fell to work, and silence ensued. But I had to stick the situation out. After all, not one of these Liver-wurst Ladies weighed less than 220 pounds; not one was over five feet, four inches tall. Here was the chance for a very candid glimpse at fat people. I just had to see my little adventure through.

Soon the liverwurst sandwiches with *no butter* were gone. Time for desserts. Said the first lady to the second lady, "And now, my dear, I'm going to make you very jealous. I'm going to have chocolate layer cake."

Said Liverwurst Lady No. 2, with a most accusing look, "Doesn't your conscience hurt you?"

"No," said No. 1. "I want it."

Up piped Liverwurst Lady No. 3 to Liverwurst Lady No. 2, "She's smart. She's getting what she wants."

The soda clerk by this time had deftly placed an enticing portion of layer cake before the beaming countenance of Liverwurst Lady No. 1. He looked at Liverwurst Lady No. 2, for all the world like a cat looking at a mouse, and said, "And yours, Madam?"

Lady No. 2 registered a stageworthy blend of agony

and wistfulness, and, with a despairing glance at the layer cake, said in a tone of complete surrender, "Oh, I'll have layer cake, too."

There was a fateful moment when the clerk, after a hasty glance at the cake shelf, said, "I'm sorry, lady, there's no more chocolate layer cake. But," he added swiftly, "we *do* have lemon and maple layer cake." From the look on the face of Lady No. 2, you would have sworn that he had saved her life.

She wasted no time. "I'll have the lemon layer cake and coffee, please."

"Oh, yes, coffee for me, too," said the first lady, "and two creams, please." Then with a sort of superior little smile on her face, she said to the other two, "I *don't* use sugar!"

The lemon layer cake was served in all its glory. The first lady had already taken a comforting mouthful of her chocolate layer cake. The lemon layer cake was about to be attacked, when the third Liverwurst Lady abjectly surrendered. She murmured, "I'll have some lemon layer cake, too."

Well, that closed the chapter as far as I was concerned. I'd bet a handsome wager that each one of those three would have been just the type to tell you, "Everything I eat turns to fat."

My thoughts wandered to Sarah, the unseen. Somewhere in that big store, Sarah was sitting, huffing and puffing, and resting the knees that hurt her. The fragments of gossip about her told her story.

There she sat, unhappily alone, no doubt wondering about her complaining knees—knees fashioned by Nature to carry a moderate weight, but now compelled to support an extra 100 pounds since Sarah had moved to Brooklyn.

Her husband, the "nice little fellow" (when they moved to Brooklyn)—just picture his unhappy plight. According to the evidence, he is a little man; undoubtedly, when he was attracted to Sarah and married her, she must have been about his size—perhaps smaller.

She was a girl with a nice figure, one that her friends still remember. We can guess that she must have weighed perhaps 120 pounds—a girl Sam liked to take to movies, to a show or a dance, a girl that he loved enough to marry, the girl that he had selected for a mate.

When they moved to Brooklyn, Sarah apparently started on the royal road to rotundity. It ended up with the gain of 100 extra pounds. Here, certainly, was a different Sarah from the one Sam had married. The girl he took to the altar had one chin; the lady he comes home to in Brooklyn now probably has three.

I hold no brief for men who neglect their wives, but Sam did not deserve the lambasting he got from the

Liverwurst Ladies. The girl he married had disappeared gradually under billowing rolls of fat. Gracious, no little man likes to walk down the street with a woman twice his size, even if she is his wife! Perhaps, in justice, the blame for that marital situation lay with Sarah, who thought so little of her husband and so much of her food that she allowed herself to grow into a waddling mountain of flesh.

That's the adventure of the Liverwurst Ladies, as I like to call it. It brings us face to face with the most difficult problem in reducing—the problem of human nature. Now bear with me a minute, please. We are not going to indulge in the overworked indoor sport of berating human nature. It is overdone these days and generally done very badly. As a matter of fact, the person who flays human nature most severely is, too often, a most flagrant example of its perversities, perplexities, and weaknesses. But we simply cannot go on until we take human nature into our reckoning.

You see, this is about as good a time as any to tell you frankly that we are in dead earnest about persuading you to reduce.

I may be a little "cracked" on the subject of the importance of health and disease. I was brought up in my father's Sanitarium, lived within its gates until my high school days. A healthy youth, a happy one, I constantly rubbed shoulders with sick people, young and old.

Just as the tenement child is intimately acquainted with the squalor and horror of poverty, so I got a first-hand view of the misery and terror of sickness and premature death. I grew up with an abiding horror of disease, and perhaps a fanatical appreciation of health.

To me, there is no more important endeavor in life than to plan, work, and aspire to live long—and to live free from the tyranny of disease. The value of health is far above that of financial achievement, social success or political freedom. After all, there is no bondage so fearful, no poverty so cruel, no failure so unhappy as that encompassed by the word *sickness*.

Perhaps this view was, unwittingly, best expressed by the wit, Ed Wynn, when he said, "What shall it profit a man if he gains the whole world and becomes the richest man in the cemetery?" When we become more wise and reasonable human beings, we shall strive to live healthfully with the same ardor and effort that we now expend in trying to outdo the Joneses.

The Grim Reaper has a thousand weapons other than the Scythe with which we usually picture him, and none is sharper or more serviceable to him than excessive obesity. We may laugh and joke with each other about fat and overweight. But Debble Fat laughs last.

The cost of overweight in human suffering and human life is impossible to calculate. I have an earnest belief that I am doing a bit of good, in a world that

39

needs a lot of good done, by helping people to reduce. But to help *you* reduce, I have to give you more than a set of diet directions; I have to help you understand fat, and fat people.

The Liverwurst Ladies can aid us. I have never forgotten them—they were examples. Those three worthies were lipophilic, no question about that, but they didn't have to be fat. They ordered, of their own will and desire, the liverwurst sandwiches and layer cake—food which just naturally spells fat to individuals constructed as they were. We can guess from their conversation that they knew very well that those foods were fattening, yet they insisted upon eating them.

I remember noting that while the three ladies were all very stout, each one conformed more or less to a certain type. The first Liverwurst Lady, I am sure, would be classed as a thyroid type of fat person; the second, as that roly-poly pituitary type; and the third leaned heavily toward what is called the maternal or ovarian type of fat.

These are technical names that you may forget now if you please, but the ladies undoubtedly had the so-called glandular types of fatness. Probably, each one of them murmured often, "I eat like a bird."

To be honest, they no doubt ate much less than they wanted. Perhaps, like many lipophilics, they were possessed of big appetites. Pity them if they were. Lipophilics with medium-sized appetites have a bad enough time of it; those with generous ones are in for double trouble.

Many a fat person eats only half of what he really wants to eat. Too bad! If he only knew, the kind—not the quantity—of the food he eats is what matters.

That skinny fellow over there likes to eat, too. And, likely as not, he eats twice as much as we do. Lipophilics have an altered body chemistry. I believe it can be made normal; certainly it can be compromised with. So while we may have to be lipophilic, we do not have to be fat.

The point is, lipophilics do not understand why they are different from the four out of five who are not lipophilic—why their eating habits have to vary from those of most people. There is the rub, and that is the gist of our story. Fat people unaware of this undeniable fact (or aware of it but unwilling to acknowledge it) fall back on excuses. That's bad!

We will not fight fat successfully with excuses, so let us dispose of these deterrents.

Generally, the excuses for being fat run in three classical patterns:

1. *It's glands!*
2. *It runs in the family!!*
3. *My work is too confining!!!*

And excuses, to paraphrase Shakespeare, make the fault of fatness all the worse by the very excuse. Since we must dissect some of them carefully, we will have to lead you into a rather strange experience—the inside story of fat people.

Have you ever noticed how a tailor or a person interested in the dress goods business casts a rather speculative eye over your clothes? I have, and I always feel a little uncomfortable. Maybe my imagination is too good.

The last cloak-and-suiter with whom I lunched had me especially worried. Mind you, not a remark passed between us about clothes or cloth, but I had the discomforting notion that he was carefully appraising the almost new suit I was wearing.

I imagined he was saying to himself, "Well, Lindlahr may know something about calories, but he doesn't know anything about clothes. Wait till the first rain hits the rags he's wearing. Strictly Grade C stuff. They will be shining like a new brass nameplate in six weeks. Probably paid a good price for them, too. It only goes to show. . . ."

Every man to his trade, I suppose. Whenever I see fat people and have a brief chance to study them, I try to size up their characters and general types. I speculate a little bit on how much they eat, and wonder what they eat, and wonder why they don't get wise to themselves and take off some of that weight.

I wonder what their fat fate is going to be. Not that I am morbid, but just as a man acquainted with details about various automobiles has a good idea of how each type will behave on the road and just about when they'll end up at the wreckers, so the person who understands fat has some idea of the general fate awaiting average fat persons, and can reflect on what the end will be.

We can learn much in the next chapter by examining the characters of some various types of lipophilics. We will be introduced, so to speak, to a few people.

Try to understand these fictional characters. And if you can find traits, habits or faults that you share with them, 'fess up. Then strengthen or oust the weak links in your character, because, they really are the villains that make you fat!

Remember the lines of Robert Burns:

> *Oh wad some power the giftie gie us*
> *To see oursels as others see us!*

CHAPTER FIVE

"It's Glands!"

JENNY WAS a nice-looking girl in her school days and after she went to work. She wasn't exactly skinny; in fact, she was quite generously rounded. Jenny knew from experience that it wasn't difficult for her to put on weight. But Jenny as a "Miss," consciously or unconsciously, refused to let pounds accumulate. Once or twice they did, quite modestly, and she set to work on them with determination. She did not allow herself to develop even a hint of obesity.

Then she won Joseph Contented. It was a good match. All the relatives approved, Joe was happy and pleased, and vistas of a nice life opened before them. Jenny had a beautiful wedding, and everyone wished the young couple luck.

A cold, calculating scientist would probably tell us that Jenny had now, in a measure, satisfied a biological urge. Perhaps Jenny wouldn't understand what that meant, but she would admit, perhaps, under cross-examination, that after she married Joe, she was not so careful about the invading pounds. It had always been an effort for her to stay slim. Now she had her man, now she had a home, now all of a sudden, it did not seem so important to deny herself the tidbits she liked to eat, or to attack savagely every extra pound that accumulated. Yes, Jenny gave up.

She relaxed her vigilance. The insidious ounces of fat accumulated, slowly and subtly, a little bit here and a little bit there, only an extra two-pieces-of-butter-and-toast's worth a day (only one ounce a day, two pounds per month). The first anniversary of her marriage spelled twenty-four pounds plus. The next celebration found her with an even larger surplus. Jenny was a nibbler and a muncher, always or almost always chewing something!

Jenny grew really heavy with the years—the moon-faced type. She developed rather serious digestive troubles. "Gall bladder," said Joe's family doctor. "Jenny has a bad thyroid gland, too. She should take thyroid tablets. . . ."

Jenny was easy-going. Too much trouble to go to doctors. Expensive, too. Then one night just two weeks before Christmas, Jenny had a gallstone attack. Very bad. Hospital . . . operation. She didn't come back.

The doctor was not surprised, for he knew that gall stones occur three times as frequently in women as they do in men. Overweight women are especially susceptible to gall bladder troubles.

Women 25 to 44 per cent over-weight had a mortality from gall bladder disease four and one-third times that of the average for the whole experience, and over ten times that of under-weight women.*

Then there was Mrs. Noah Illusions. She had the same tendency toward fat that Jenny Contented possessed. However, Mrs. Noah loved her husband enough to curb her appetite and watch her diet.

But Noah turned out to be a bad husband who shattered all his wife's dreams. He neglected her, chased around with other women. He failed utterly to respond to her earnest efforts at homemaking.

For a time bewildered, Mrs. Noah didn't quite comprehend. She tried desperately to win his companionship and strengthen marital ties. She failed. Finally she gave up; she couldn't win.

Mrs. Noah was not the type to repay Noah in kind. She could not be unfaithful as he was. She couldn't take to drink. It was impossible for her to express frustration in any immoral way (by ordinary stand-

*"Build of Women and Its Relation to Their Mortality— A Preliminary Report," Louis I. Dublin and Herbert H. Marks, Metropolitan Life Insurance Company, *Proceedings of Association of Life Insurance Medical Directors of America,* 1938.

ards). So she sank gradually into gluttony, indulging her appetite for foods—rich foods, fattening foods. Eating gave her an escape. She took solace in reading—and nibbled candy with every chapter. She just loved butter.

Mrs. Noah brooded and breaded. Ten years later, she grew very sick. High blood pressure and bad arteries, said the doctor.

The internes at the hospital where she went for observation nudged each other and exclaimed over her fat. What a build, said they, and with true professional interest classed her as a pituitary type.

The doctor discussed her case at staff meeting. A terrific blood pressure, with fat undoubtedly a contributing factor. He added:

High blood pressure is found more frequently in women because there are more fat women. The extra weight causes a premature breakdown of the circulatory system.

The mortality figures are as follows:

DISEASES OF THE ARTERIES DEATH RATE PER 100,000*
Normal Weight	Overweight		
	5%–14%	15%–24%	25% plus
23	34	46	41 †

*"The Influence of Weight on Certain Causes of Death," (*Human Biology,* issue of May, 1930) by Louis I. Dublin,

Interesting, too, is the case of Mrs. Materna Tee, five feet two. Before her baby came, she was on the slim side, with lovely curves. However, when she was carrying her baby, she began to put on weight. Her doctor insisted upon her eating plenty of nourishing food. He was an ardent advocate of the time-worn adage, "The pregnant woman must eat for two."

Materna was carefully instructed to take things easy and to eat good, rich, nourishing food. The advice was

Metropolitan Life Insurance Company, with the collaboration of Herbert H. Marks.

All the statistics quoted in Chapters 5, 6, and 15 on the death rates for certain diseases among overweight individuals as compared with those among individuals of normal weight are taken, with the author's permission, from the above source.

The statistics were compiled from records of 192,304 white men insured by the Union Central Life Insurance Company during the years 1887 to 1908. These men, all examined by physicians and found free from organic diseases or serious impairments at the time the insurance was placed, were traced from the time the insurance was issued until the policy anniversary in 1921 or earlier termination of the insurance.

Since the first four years of experience were discounted, the effect was to offset effects of medical selection and to limit the study to men of 20 years of age or over. The total picture is based on 1,487,561 life years. As the men were of a comparatively high economic standard and were not employed in hazardous occupations, the rates are all the more impressive. Deaths in the group during the observation period numbered 13,350.

†Diminishes because apoplexy and cerebral hemorrhage get them first.

not unpleasant to follow. The fifth month of her pregnancy, she was eating three meals of plentiful proportions a day; cookies and cakes and odds and ends of food were an increasing indulgence between meals. She could put away a box of vanilla wafers and two glasses of milk before she retired for bed, and each month found her growing fatter and fatter until the ninth month showed a net gain of thirty pounds in weight.

No one in her circle of acquaintances was particularly surprised; in fact, they rather expected that Materna would grow fat. "Babies do that," they said. "It's ovaries!"

Mr. Tee was solicitous and kind and beamed approvingly at Materna's progress. Finally the day arrived. Materna had a bad time of it. The ten and one-half pound baby came with difficulty, and complications followed. In after years, the eating habits she had acquired as an expectant mother never left her. When other babies came, her weight increased. "It's my glands," she would explain—over a banana split.

One day she was struck by a car and severely bruised. The hospital doctors found that she had Bright's disease.

While we know that obesity predisposes mightily toward kidney disease, it is a strange circumstance that

pedestrian accident rates are also higher among overweights (especially women):

ACUTE AND CHRONIC NEPHRITIS DEATH RATE PER 100,000

Normal Weight		Overweight	
	5%–14%	15%–24%	25% plus
82	108	202	224

ACCIDENT DEATH RATE PER 100,000

Normal Weight		Overweight	
60	65	65	87

It is true that overweight is divided according to medical textbooks into two general types, one called exogenous, the other endogenous. These are $25 words. Exogenous fat is caused by eating more fattening food than the body requires; the endogenous type is supposed to be largely due to disturbances of one or another of the internal secretory glands.

Various authorities have estimated that the exogenous (eating incorrectly) types of fat comprise from 95 to 98 per cent of all cases of overweight—not much of an excuse for the conscience of that 260-pound Mrs. Ohno Nottme who blissfully enjoys a double chocolate ice cream soda with whipped cream.

Yes, the glandular theory of fat has lulled many a conscience to sleep. "It's my glands, dearie. Everything I eat turns to fat."

Oh, my, what a comfort that premise is. Many a

good soul has resigned completely in the fight against fat because of that profundity, and waxed fatter and fatter with the years. But, sad to say, it is not quite the truth. Here is a definition from Dorland's *Medical Dictionary*: endogenous obesity—"obesity due to a combination of overeating and metabolic (endocrine [glandular]) abnormalities." Note the word "combination."

Here is what usually happens. Inefficient glands do not produce obesity. It's the other way around—obesity produces inefficient glands. After a person has eaten, for too many years, too big a percentage of fattening foods, the glands which regulate the metabolism of this sort of food get out of kilter.

Loading the body with excesses of fattening foods may begin in babyhood. It may commence even before the baby is born, as the developing baby-to-be is conditioned by the mother's blood. If this is overcharged with fattening foods, the baby's fat and starch food metabolism makes a bad start.

Every class of food has its own specially designed reception in the body. Sugars, starches and fats, which are the fattening foods, each have a special metabolism. Fat metabolism includes team work by the liver, pancreas, intestines, lymph glands, and internal secretory glands such as the thyroid, pituitary, and ovaries. Body mechanisms can stand much abuse. However,

51

there are costs, and if involved organs, tissues, and other structures of the body are forced to accommodate themselves to an abnormal process, they must rearrange their functions or forms to meet its demands. That is why a toe dancer's leg muscles may overdevelop, or why a workingman's hands may grow large and horny.

And so, when a person punishes and overworks the fat-regulating functions, these may become abnormal. The glands involved get out of order. As a result, the fat person in time may begin to develop a peculiar shape; excess fat may deposit in the body middle and form a paunch, or distribute itself here, there, and elsewhere in the body in certain patterns.

The doctor who greets the patient for the first time in his office often can take one look and say, "Well, you have a thyroid fat," or "You have a pituitary fat." If it isn't readily apparent which particular type of fat the victim has developed, the doctor can conveniently and correctly say, "Well, all your glands are out of order. You have a pluri-glandular type of fat."

Yes, in time most of us fatties develop some glandular type of fat. No doubt about that. But the internal secretory glands are not the culprits—they are victims. An unhappy choice of eating has hurt them.

CHAPTER SIX

"It Runs in the Family"

THAT LAST CHAPTER was rather unkind to the ladies. It was unfair, because men are far more apt to make excuses for fat than their sisters. "I come by it honestly," they say. "It runs in the family," and/or "My work is too confining."

Stanislaus Mutcheat, the butcher, and his brothers Alex the baker and Louie the candlestick maker, all weighed over 220 pounds. Big men, the Mutcheats. Stan weighed 240. His father had been a big man, too. His mother, five feet three, weighed 197 when she passed on.

Back in the days when the Mutcheat family graced the Snorkle Benevolent Brotherhood picnics, they were an eye-filling sight. Said many a good soul to another when the Mutcheats lumbered by, "Wow! Fat certainly runs in that family. Look at them! They're all fat!"

Of course they were. But, we pray you, look at what they ate. Papa Mutcheat always liked fatty, greasy dishes and plenty of bread and potatoes. He drank beer with his meals. Mrs. Mutcheat fixed them for him because she wanted to please her husband. She weighed only 115 pounds when they were married, but she gained fifteen pounds the first year, and she reached 175 before Stan graduated from grammar school. She usually ate a bite of breakfast with each one of the boys, and was likely to sample her own cooking quite frequently.

As for the boys—well, babies are not born with a taste for foods. They develop tastes. The kind of food that is served in the home will largely determine what the children learn to like.

What kind of food do you suppose the Mutcheat boys learned to like? Spinach? No. They usually ate meat, potatoes, and pie, and plenty of them. They were the big jam and bread and butter boys too, in grammar school. When he grew to manhood, Stan used to order double portions of the meat dish at lunch rooms. "A big guy like me has got to eat." He always had peanuts in his pockets. Customers at the store used to look at his expansive stomach and say, "It's a good thing you own this place." And Stan would beam approvingly.

If someone had told Stan that fat is not hereditary—that it is an acquired characteristic—he would have shrugged his shoulders and said "Yeah?"

Pressed to debate the proposition, he probably would

have agreed that you don't build fat out of your ancestors. He would have agreed, too, that his grandparents didn't order meals for him—and so, perhaps, he was a right reasonable human being.

Stan took a partner the year after he developed diabetes. A sixteen-hour day was too much for him. In the back of the diabetic manual the doctor gave him were some statements:

DIABETES DEATH RATE PER 100,000

Normal Weight	Overweight		
	5%–14%	15%–24%	25% plus
14	22	45	117

(More than 78% of diabetic men are overweight—women, 83%.)

Stan figured that was the doctor's concern.

"My fat is hereditary." Well, I could use that excuse. My father was five feet seven and one-half inches tall, and in the late 1890's weighed 278 pounds.

My very fat paternal grandfather died in 1881 at the age of 51 of cerebral apoplexy. Our family history relates that my grandfather's father was fat. If fat ever runs in families, it runs in mine.

Shame on my ancestors for sending my weight up to 207 that summer at Juan-les-Pins. But what has happened to these ghosts since then? I weigh thirty-one pounds less. Perhaps my meals had something to do with it. Fat is built from what we eat.

55

John Gettingon was a grammar school mate of Stan's, but he had gone on to high school and college. When he started with the Suxess Corporation, he was lean and rangy. John was a "comer." He worked hard —his energy pace was terrific. Before many seasons passed, John was made sales manager.

As he divested himself of detail and sat long in conferences, he grew less and less active. Five years later, his major work was to help direct policies and shape the course of the business.

The driving urge that once tempered him like fine steel relaxed. John Gettingon grew satisfied. He had not only the means but also the time to eat more. He liked a comforting midnight supper—it helped him to sleep. John gradually developed paunch, haunch, and jowls.

First he greeted his accumulating fat as becoming to his dignity and position. Later, when he hit 190, he joined a gym club (to which he never found time to go). He joined a golf club, too, but his game wasn't so good, so he would dub around for a few holes and then play bridge at the clubhouse.

When he passed the 210-pound mark, John took the gentle ribbing of his friends quite seriously. "Yes, I am overweight. Not enough exercise. I could work this fat off in no time if I didn't have to keep my nose to the grindstone."

John finally developed heart disease and had to resign. Musing about it, his fellow directors concluded that while John's heart trouble seemed to come very suddenly, it must have been developing for some time.

Yes, come to think of it, John had been slowing up for quite a while. Seems as if the company could have done better these last few years. Maybe it wasn't breaks alone that sent the New Company sales ahead of theirs. . . . Yes, John had been sick and hadn't told them. That was it, and just like him—stout fellow.

Yet Shakespeare said: "Fat paunches have lean pates; and dainty bits make rich the ribs, but banker out the wits."

Meanwhile, John mourned the day when he had allowed himself to get so fat that he could not qualify for insurance. There was the mortgage—and he hadn't saved much.

The insurance company had turned him down on the authority of cold figures:

ORGANIC HEART DISEASE RATE PER 100,000

Normal Weight	Overweight		
	5%–14%	15%–24%	25% plus
80	115	135	129*

*The apparent drop in death rate among those 25% overweight is largely due to the fact that angina pectoris, apoplexy—"sudden death"—take their lives. The death rate for angina pectoris doubles for overweights.

57

That wail—"I don't get enough exercise"—is such a lame excuse for obesity.

Exercise does firm the tissues and trim down the contours of the body. It helps to get rid of droopiness and flabbiness which exaggerate the appearance of fat. But the chap who bewails the fact that he can't exercise enough is *not* exercising enough, and that's the rub. His chances of doing so are cut from the same cloth as those day dreams wherein he fondly imagines that someday he *will* exercise. He can have absolutely no conception of the tremendous amount of exercise needed to burn a bit of fat.

To take weight down via exercise is to choose the hard way. It is the most difficult and unsatisfactory method of getting rid of a pound of fat. A 200-pound man, for example, would have to play handball furiously for almost six hours really to burn up a pound of body fat. Though he might sweat two pounds of perspiration from his body in the game, this is not losing fat.

Call it laziness if you will, but personally I would rather pass up two slices of bread at a meal than put myself under the energy-expense obligations involved. At my weight, it would take an hour of brisk walking to use up the equivalent of two pieces of bread and butter. That is too much trouble.

Stubborn stuff, that LARD we call body fat. The

overweight gymnasium boys fool themselves by forgetting that perspiration accounts for most of the weight they apparently lose at the gym. It is easy to sweat out from a pound to three pounds of water with exercise. Drinking water puts it back. Exercise sharpens the appetite, too. Those slim, trim athletic chaps who attribute their lack of obesity to exercise are not true lipophilics. They would never be really fat. They are among the four (lucky devils) out of five.

But most important of all, do you remember Lavoisier and that physiological entity, the metabolism rate? Remember how it goes down as we grow older? Well, if you would like to know the reasons, scientific and factual, translated into terms of exercise versus fat, here is how it would work out (please understand this is the roughest kind of approximation):

If, with all factors such as food intake, occupation, and environment being equal, a man at the age of 20 could maintain his weight by playing fourteen holes of golf three times a week, at 30 he would have to play fifteen to accomplish the same result. At 40, our active friend would have to play sixteen holes to preserve the status quo. It would require seventeen holes at 50, and eighteen at 60. In short, the older he grew, the more he would have to exercise. Yet it is obvious that the older the man, the less able he is to exercise. Also the fatty gets caught in a vicious circle;

fat discourages activity. To put it simply, the fatter a man gets, the lazier he grows. The lazier he is, the fatter he becomes.

If the lipophilic will but remember that exercise of a little judgment in selecting foods is the best exercise of all, he will do much better. A fatty piece of roast beef with greasy gravy—in comparison with a lean piece of the same meat without gravy—obligates a 200 pound man to something like nine holes of golf over an average course. I will take the food way to slimness.

Yes, it is how you exercise your knife and fork that counts the most. As some wit once put it, the best exercise in the world for a fat person is to stop abruptly in the middle of a meal, place his hands on the edge of the table and push his chair away. With that, he gets up and walks to another room.

That is a simple little exercise. It requires only half a minute to execute, and it is the most efficient reducing exercise you'll ever find.

Hardly an excuse is the loud boast of George Begay, the big butter-and-egg man. A good earner, big spender, and darling of night clubs everywhere. He has tremendous energy—can put in a night of roistering and apparently do two men's work the next day.

George likes to eat much and drink more. He holds his liquor well, and takes an inordinate pride in his eating. He likes to astonish people with the amount of food he can consume. A daily total of 4000 calories of food and 3000 calories' worth of alcohol is not unusual with him.

It is true he uses up a terrific amount of energy—perhaps double the amount that you and I do. Still that is only an extra 2500 calories' worth—which still allows him to gain weight at an alarming pace. (Only 100 unneeded calories per day—a cocktail, an extra piece of toast, etc.—mean a pound gained each month, twelve pounds a year, a hundred pounds in nine years.)

George has a marvelous disposition, a wonderful sense of humor, and a heart of gold, as the saying goes. It seems to be no trouble for him to land big orders from his customers. They like him, and like to throw business his way.

But George weighs over 300 pounds, and his weight seems to be going up and up. This tendency frightens some of his very best friends, and they remonstrate with him.

"Listen," says George. "With me, it's a short life and a merry one. If I have to go out like a light some day, okay. I've lived well, I've done whatever I wanted to do, and I've had as much fun in almost any one day of my life as the average guy has in a week."

A short life and a merry one. It's a philosophy that might have some justice to it if it would work accord-

61

ing to plan. I suppose the George Begays know very well that they are virtually killing themselves. Doctors warn them of their blood pressure, tell them that the big, florid, heavy type of fellow is peculiarly subject to apoplexy. The Georges may even be familiar with these figures:

CEREBRAL HEMORRHAGE AND APOPLEXY DEATH
RATE PER 100,000

Normal Weight	Overweight		
	5%–14%	15%–24%	25% plus
70	101	115	170

"But," they say, "it's not a bad way to go. Presto! Something snaps, then you're through." What they don't know is that the majority of men who have apoplectic strokes do not "go out like a light." One, two or ten years of a really tragic existence may follow.

You will see these prophets of a short life and a merry one helpless with paralysis in a wheelchair. You will wonder, sadly, what thoughts go on in their minds. Here are those who loved life dearly—the good times, jolly companions, and all the amusements the hail-fellow-well-met lives for. It is a cruel punishment that glues them in a chair where they must sit helpless and useless and watch life all about them.

The short life and the merry one is utterly impossible to ordain. Probably, fourteen times out of fifteen, the chronic degenerative disease that is brought about by high living involves long torture. It seems as if Providence were strict about paying the George Begays on the basis of an eye for an eye and a tooth for a tooth.

It just doesn't work out.

Such are a few of the excuses for tolerating obesity. It is almost unbelievable what self-deception fat people can practice. Honest mistakes are made, of course. Many mothers gain many pounds while nursing their babies because of the false notion that they have to eat *rich* foods. They need, instead, the mineral and vitamin foods, which are not fattening.

Many people develop fat after an operation or during convalescence. They of course do not know that the metabolism rate goes down when we are inactive. Fat accumulates more readily then, and we should eat *less* fattening foods. Weight sometimes piles on after the forties, because of the much lower metabolism after the change, which both men and women go through.

When body fat begins to accumulate, eating habits must be changed. Circumstances may make lipophilics out of those who once were not. However, most people delude themselves about how much they eat—as far as trying to watch their diet is concerned, they postpone action deliberately. They are afraid their appetites and comfort will be assailed if they try to take off weight.

63

That, good reader, is not true. It is a misconception bred by ignorance of foods. It signifies an utter lack of knowledge about foods. It is a mistake which we can correct.

CHAPTER SEVEN

Events That Cast Shadows

TODAY I am introduced on the radio as a nutritionist and an authority on reducing. Why? It has deep roots, that claim, for in reality it goes back to my father's youth.

My father was educated to be a plant brewing and baking chemist, but in the early 1880's, like many another young man in those days, he went west. He drifted into business, buying and selling land in tempo with the advancing railroads.

Finally, Kalispell, Montana, caught his fancy, particularly because he met my mother there. He married and settled down when he was close to 40—a typical John Gettingon.

Men lived well and ate well in those roistering days of a burly young West. At the time of his marriage, Henry Lindlahr weighed over 250 pounds, and considered a brace of ducks a fine appetizer for a hearty meal.

A few years later, he developed diabetes of the serious type, and began the rounds. There were some

65

spectacular treatments for diabetes in those days. One of the well known doctors of the day put Father on a ham and champagne diet.

His condition grew worse. Advised, finally, to settle his affairs, he disposed of his business interest, and the year 1898 saw my mother, him, and me en route for Vienna.

Various treatments and "cures" at different spas proved unavailing; Father made his peace with God and prepared to die. Then, through the importunities of a boyhood chum, he was persuaded to try the services of a famous natural healer—Father Kneipp. Father Kneipp had no medical training, but in his world-famous clinic at Woerishofen, Bavaria, he prescribed the water cure, strict dieting and other natural methods of treatment—with eminent success.

My father had absolutely no faith in the idea that a natural healer could help him. He went to Woerishofen only to satisfy his friend.

He had to wait ten days for his appointment with Father Kneipp. He heard wondrous stories of the spectacular cures of this priest who leaned on Nature for his methods. He met patients who were healed of so-called incurable ailments—healed with *diet*, baths, sunshine, and strict living. Remember, doctors practiced very differently in those days from the way they do now. Those years were the peak of that fantastic era in medical practice when doctors gave from one to three drugs for every symptom (poly-pharmacy).

Finally it was Father's turn for consultation with the healer.

He received a shock when he stepped up for his few allotted minutes with the water cure priest. Father Kneipp took a searching look at him, asked to smell his breath, and then said: "You are *pig* [glutton]. You eat too much. You are too fat. You have the sugar disease. You will take sitz baths and live on fruits and greens and vegetables alone. No bread, no cereals, no meats, no alcohol of any kind. See Sister Celeste."

Sister Celeste, one of Father Kneipp's assistants, gave my father full details of his strict diet regimen. Of course it is no miracle to us, in the light of modern knowledge, that a strict fruit and vegetable diet would rid a patient of excess sugar in the blood and its symptoms. It is readily understandable now, but in those days of plain and fancy futile treatments for diabetes, a no-medicine treatment that really worked was startling!

Springtime greeted a new Henry Lindlahr. His sugar was gone. He had lost over forty pounds. His life had been saved.

We came back to America. But something else had happened to Father. Business no longer held an interest for him. The miracle of diet absorbed him, body and

67

soul. He mourned that his fat father might yet have been alive had he been told how to eat. He had lost a fat sister before she reached 30. He had seen loved friends die, and from what little he knew then, he suspected that some of them might have been saved if they had been told how to eat. A John Gettingon had faced death long months; he saw life in a new perspective.

In short, Henry Lindlahr became a full-fledged diet enthusiast. He was restive, burning with new resolves. He wanted to help other people. He must. Finally he made up his mind to study medicine.

Father was graduated in 1904. While the medical schools of the day had no courses in nutrition and dietetics, Father had left no page unturned in the lore of foods and diet.

He pored over the writings of Hippocrates, who had used the livers of birds and animals to cure night blindness and certain inflammatory diseases of the eyes. He marvelled over the discoveries of Lind of Great Britain, who had advised Captain Cook to carry sauerkraut and lemons on his ships to cure the sailors of scurvy. He learned how rice hulls cured beriberi. He studied diet, diet, diet.

So he accumulated a store of knowledge, some of it exact and scientific, some of it based upon folklore and tradition, but all of it pertaining to foods and their healing virtues.

As a result, when he opened his office at 232 South Michigan Avenue, Chicago (where the Congress Hotel Annex now stands), he knew much about diet—far more than any other doctor of his time, I am sure. Within a few months he was very busy, really helping his patients with knowledge many of his medical colleagues did not possess.

In 1905 he bought a large house on Ashland Boulevard and Harrison Street, and began the Lindlahr Sanitarium. There he used his diet ideas and knowledge with such skill that his institution became eminently successful, although he never did win the approval of the medical profession.

He passed on in 1924. I wish he had lived a little longer. He would have seen diet grow into a science. He would have seen a hundred or more of the beliefs and rules of practice that he had espoused taken out of the empirical and proven by scientific facts.

He would have seen medical journals literally filled with articles on diet, vitamins, and food minerals. He would have seen the Nobel Prize awarded upon two occasions to nutritionists. He would have been tremendously pleased, for the development of nutritional science within the last few years has vindicated him, stamped him as a wise man, a good doctor—too advanced for his times.

As you can surmise, I grew up in a little world that revolved around nutrition, foods, and the treatment of disease by diet. Perhaps we had better explain that nutrition is defined as the sum total of all the physical and chemical reactions involved in the growth, repair, and maintenance of the body tissues and their proper functioning.

Essentially, there is considerable difference between a dietitian and a nutritionist. A nutritionist is concerned with the science of nutrition; a dietitian with the practical application thereof.

The summer of 1914 found me enjoying a happy vacation in nearby Michigan. I planned to sail for Europe in the Fall to enter the University of Heidelberg. The following summer I was to spend in the sanitarium of Bircher-Benner, a leading European nutritionist. We had mapped out four years of work that would encompass studies during vacations at the leading nutrition centers of the continent.

The cataclysmic upheaval in Europe, that tragic summer, put an end to my father's cherished plans for me. We cast about for an American equivalent. However, no United States medical college at that time had a course in dietetics—not one.

The only school where I could get any semblance of

a course in dietetics was the Chicago College of Osteopathy, and there I enrolled in September 1914.

The following year I took additional courses at the Jenner Medical College to earn credits toward my doctorate in medicine.

In 1918 I was graduated and licensed as an osteopathic physician and surgeon. My first few years of sanitarium practice were punctuated by jaunts here and there to take special courses relating to nutrition.

Meanwhile, I finished my medical studies. In 1923, I was graduated as a doctor of medicine. Always, always during those years, the kindly counsel and heartfelt teachings of my father were constant accompaniments of my formal studies, his vast experience in diet therapy a golden stream of knowledge for me to tap.

When I succeeded my father, the Sanitarium had been established for nineteen years. The patrons had become a pretty well-defined class—chiefly cases that could be helped by diet. A good many of them were diabetics. I had four years of practice among this group before the advent of insulin; four years, at least, of first-hand knowledge of diet as it concerned this particular ailment. It was marvelous training, I assure you, as a prelude to understanding the dietetic problems of reducing—for the nutrition problems are much the same.

71

Our diabetic diet, like any good diet for this disease, was composed mainly of low starch and low sugar vegetables and fruits. The L. C. diet, we called it (low carbohydrate).

We noted, as anyone who sees many diabetic cases will note, that most diabetics are fat, that most of them eat too much. We suspected that overeating and obesity were perhaps important causative factors. One thing was certain: we could not escape observing the steady and spectacular loss of weight sustained by fat diabetics who were placed on the L. C. diet.

I can well remember the terror of some of the relatives who visited fat diabetics under our care. Often one of them would come to me or to one of the house physicians with fear in her voice: "Oh, doctor, my husband has lost fifteen pounds in the two weeks since he has been here."

We were finally forced to explain that, in a degree, the essential part of our treatment was to take off some of the burdening pounds which we were sure had a chemical rôle in producing the ailment. That served to reassure the patients, and thus we went on, year after year, employing a diet which took weight, almost like magic, from patients on whom it was used.

Also, during all this time, there were occasions in the management of certain ailments when we prescribed what is termed a fast. The harsher name for it is starvation. A patient on a Lindlahr fast received a quart of fruit juices a day, and all the water he desired to drink, but no other food, liquid or solid, was allowed.

In the few types of sickness where this drastic treatment was indicated, it really worked marvelously well. Usually we employed only short fasts, although some of our patients would occasionally fast ten days, or, very rarely, a few days longer.

All of this is important to remember, for time finally brought this startling fact to the fore: *A person on an L. C. diet lost weight more quickly than one who was fasting.*

It is easy to write that axiom now, but with us I am afraid it had accumulated the contempt bred by familiarity. Not until 1925 did the significance of that simple rule, in so far as it relates to the reducing diet, dawn upon me.

Then in the early part of August 1925, a portly and prominent socialite from Philadelphia arrived at my Chicago office. She was most impressive and exceedingly "important." In fact, she demanded a suite of rooms, which was startling as we had been overcrowded for years and were fortunate to have a single room vacant. Yet despite our limited accommodations, she remained.

Her next act to outrage our routine was to inform me, at our preliminary meeting, that she was not sick.

73

Furthermore, she did not "see the need" of going through the regular and thorough examination which we always insisted upon. Here I disagreed, and told her rather firmly that we were not operating a hotel.

Then she told me that she had come to us to reduce. She wanted to lose thirty pounds in thirty days. With an airy wave of the hand, she said she was sure we could accomplish this feat because she knew we had had much experience with fasting. She was determined to starve to lose weight.

It developed that she was to be married in a little over a month, and wanted to look extra nice at her wedding. Also, her future husband had intimated that she was a bit overweight.

This was the first time in our experience that anything of this sort had happened. But as the lady weighed 240 pounds, I saw no harm in the idea. A thirty-pound loss for her promised benefit—and there was Dan Cupid to consider.

The Philadelphia matron began her carefully supervised fast. Seven days passed with the net result that she lost about four pounds. On the seventh day, when she happened to be on my list of calls, the interview could have been best described by the title of that Broadway hit, *Hellzapoppin*.

She expressed exceeding displeasure over her lack of progress. I suggested that she exercise a little patience, and retreated from the august presence a bit uncomfortable over the situation. In a way, I considered the whole affair a silly one. I had more important cases on hand than reducing. But by this time, the eyes of all the other patients were on Mrs. Bucks, as the nurses called her. I did some thinking.

A great light dawned on me. The L. C. diet—of course our L. C. diet took off pounds more rapidly than a fast. Actually there is a similarity between the problems of sugar chemistry in diabetes and fat chemistry in obesity, so I took that liberty and license a physician must sometimes take—to fib a bit with honorable intention—and stopped back to see the lady from Philadelphia.

I told her that I had been thinking over her progress very seriously. Her blood sugar examination would be made in the morning, to reconcile with her metabolism test, and if my suspicions were correct, I would put her on a diet which I was sure would definitely reduce her at the pound-a-day rate she had expected from a fast.

The next morning, a blood sugar test was made. It was normal, but beginning that night, the lady from the City of Brotherly Love went on our L. C. diet. She lost twelve pounds the first week, eight pounds the second, and a little over six the third.

She left for Philadelphia happy, bestowing a shower of blessings on me and handsome tips on the nurses

75

and attendants. A bit later, she sent a note to report that she had remained on the diet until her wedding day—and had lost thirty-four pounds. From that time on, she passed from my ken. Perhaps, who knows, she will read these lines. May she forgive my flippancy— she taught me a wonderful lesson.

CHAPTER EIGHT

A Great Mystery Is Solved

AFTER THE LADY from Philadelphia left, I really gave thought to the strange paradox that a person eating two and one-half to three pounds of food per day on our L. C. diet lost more weight, and lost it more consistently, than the person who was starved—the person on a fast.

I had my secretary cull out, from treatment records of the past twelve months, the histories of patients who had been on a fast (they numbered 152) and on the L. C. diet (206). Yes, the rule held.

Some questions still remained in my mind, so I detailed our junior dietitian to correlate, catalogue, and summarize for me the weight charts from January 1921 to the time of my study. Although the house physicians were supposed to keep detailed and exact progress records, quite a few cases had to be discarded in our survey because of careless entries. Nevertheless, this fact stuck out like the Empire State building: the L. C. diet was more "reducing" than a fast!

Naturally, we compared patients of approximately

the same weight. It became apparent that the greater the accumulation of body fat, the greater weight loss ratio in the L. C. group.

Please note that our fasts were not complete starvation. Diluted fruit juices staved off starvation toxemia. (Besides withdrawal of food, the actual sickness— toxemia or mild fever—produced by starvation causes some weight loss.)

A fasting patient somewhat active and free from starvation toxemia lost about three-fourths of a pound a day (2500 calories). The average weight loss on the Lindlahr seven-day reducing diet, *all cases combined,* has been over a pound a day. Heavyweights lose a pound and one-half or so daily. The same heavyweights starving (without toxemia) would probably lose only three-fourths to one pound a day (actual energy expenditure).

Now the study had become deeply interesting. Established assumptions in dietetic practice were being given a rude jolt. Fond dietetic beliefs were shattered, and established nutritional principles branded mistakes. I had to look for explanations.

The story of my subsequent search would likely be of great interest to a nutritionist, but to the lay reader it would be a dull maze of mystifying words and phrases. Here was a problem not to be solved with test tubes and guinea pigs; here was a principle to be ferreted out.

The trail led through a wilderness of what we don't know about food metabolism. I had to back-track to the study of how foods behave when burned in calorimeters. I had to seek every last morsel of knowledge about the behavior of nitrogen and the mineral elements in foods during metabolism.

The complex problems of what is called the respiratory quotient in food chemistry gave a light. The intricate workings of the water metabolism of the body gave more clues. Strangely enough, the best clue came from following the steps by which a cow makes cream out of grass.

I had to reclassify foods. Standard textbooks still apply the term carbohydrate (starch) to lettuce, mushrooms, and half a hundred other foods which have more water content than milk, and very little starch and sugar. The fact that some chapters in our established works on food chemistry should be rewritten may not seem of moment to lay readers. However, it is important, for the L. C. diet destroys fat, and the how and why is an open sesame to combating overweight.

Read carefully now—for to control body fat as easily and pleasantly as I do, you will have to take a little dip into food chemistry. The high points follow:

79

Lavoisier, remember, taught us that food produces heat in the body. What he could not discover with his head cut off, other men did.

A contemporary of Lavoisier's, swashbuckling Count Rumford (born Ben Thomson near Woburn, Massachusetts, in 1753), had invented an instrument to measure heat—the calorimeter.

To estimate heat values accurately, a specified unit of heat was devised and called a calorie, just as you call a certain amount of water a pint, or a definite unit of flour or rice an ounce.

Therefore, since Rumford's time, scientists have been busy measuring the heat-giving value of foods, and expressing it as so many calories. With this knowledge, we can reckon that a strip of bacon may give you enough body heat to work up a fine fervor in a political argument—two stalks of celery, enough coolness to snub a banker.

Many years after Rumford, a precocious and fussy Englishman, James Prescot Joule, demonstrated (in 1843, when he was 25 years old) that mechanical force has its exact equivalent in heat. Thus, a calorie of heat is also a definite measurement of energy, and we can surmise that the heat which fevers a lover's brow can also propel his legs—if an irate parent shouts "Get out!"

Two years after Joule's amazing contribution to

science, a stiff-necked Prussian out of Potsdam, Hermann Ludwig Ferdinand von Helmholtz, proved that any form of energy can be transformed into another—and that the sum total of all energy in the universe is constant.

We find, then, by applying this law, that some curves of a double chin may be just a locked-up ten-mile walk. Thus, if you are in the mood to dispense with a fold or two, you can do so by undertaking a vigorous hike. The energy you use is provided by burning up body fat. (Let's hope it comes from the chin deposits).

Now, to recapitulate: Body energy and heat are supplied by foods. Heat and energy not used are stored as fat. It follows that if we lipophilics eat more fat-forming food than we can use, the surplus will be stored as fat, perhaps jowls, or an extra bulge in the abdomen.

All of this does not explain why my patients, eating three pounds of food a day on the L. C. diet, lost more weight than those who were fasting.

Here is the answer to the puzzle, as simply as I can state it.

It costs body heat and energy to digest food. When you eat a piece of steak, your teeth must grind it. Esophageal muscles carry the chewed morsels to your stomach, where they are rocked to and fro for a few

81

hours, while little glands provide ferments which partly digest them.

Later, thirty-three feet of intestines will mold and enfold what was once a steak, and a few other digestive juices will change the material into more simple chemical forms.

Finally, tiny suction pumps will carry some of the digested steak to lymph glands in your body for further use. Blood cells will patiently load a microscopic bit into their hollows, and carry it to hungry cells throughout the body.

The liver, the spleen and the pancreas will play a part in this process. The heart will beat harder for it. Even the lungs will take in more air because you have eaten a steak. All told, you use a considerable amount of body heat and energy (calories) in this complicated process of chewing and digesting a piece of steak, and assimilating its ultimate fractions for body use.

There is no way to calculate, in exact calorie value, the amount of heat and energy a given person will use in metabolizing a piece of steak. The calorie cost will vary with the individual, for we all behave just a little bit differently.

We do know, however, that it does not require nearly as much body energy to digest the steak as the steak itself will provide. We make an energy (calorie) profit out of the transaction.

To illustrate: A four-ounce piece of steak may supply about 200 calories. If we assume, for the sake of simplicity, that the average person uses about twenty-five calories of body energy preparing this steak for body use, he will make a net profit of 175 calories. If these are used up in exercise, work, sleep or play, good enough. If not, they may be stored as an ounce of fat.

Now let us consider the metabolic fate of four ounces of spinach. All those processes involved in the digestion of a piece of steak must also take place to digest a portion of spinach. The same whirling and twirling of the digestive system, the same physical and chemical commotion—there is not much difference. The metabolic heat cost and body energy expense in digesting four ounces of spinach is as great as in digesting four ounces of steak.

In fact, the calorie cost in spinach digestion may be greater, owing to its relatively high mineral value and roughage content. (There is practically no metabolic cost in digesting sugar and alcohol—remember that.)

Four ounces of cooked spinach will yield seventeen calories of energy value. If we use the same arbitrary figure that we did with steak, and allow twenty-five calories of energy and heat to digest the spinach, we find that the spinach eater would lose heat and energy, in the transaction, to the extent of eight calories.

Where are these extra calories of energy to come

from? The body cannot find them in the spinach, so they must come eventually from stored fat in the body.

That is why eating spinach alone would cause an actual weight (calorie) loss to the body. There are many foods of the same nature. Obviously, they come in very handy for reducing diets.

After I arrived at this fundamental fact in the metabolic behavior of certain foods, a convenient term to designate them as a class was needed. I chose "catabolic foods" as a logical name.

Body metabolism is composed of two separate divisions of activity: one is the breaking down of tissues, called catabolism; the other is the building up of tissues, called anabolism. In youth the body grows and develops; anabolism is then greater than catabolism.

When foods create a deficit in the body fat, they may properly be called catabolic foods because the process of losing weight is a catabolic process. Adding fat to the body is an anabolic process and foods which will perform this function may be called the anabolic foods.

After growth has been completed, anabolism and catabolism remain equal; the body tissues retain a status quo as far as growth is concerned. In the later years of life, the catabolic processes increase, the tissues shrink, and the weight grows less.

Generally speaking, the person who puts on extra fat is receiving too generous treatment from the anabolic processes. If anabolism could be tamed down some and remain equal to catabolism, body weight would stay at a normal level. This is just what happens with many fortunate people.

It is desirable for the overweight person to have an increase in catabolism until the weight becomes normal.

When we found that some foods were definitely catabolic, we found excellent weapons to regulate metabolism. Our next step was to study foods and class them as *anabolic* and *catabolic*, as the case might be. At first glance, it might seem strange that some foods really take weight from the body, but when the facts are appreciated, it is understandable, for some foods have a very specific purpose in nutrition. They supply rare but vitally needed minerals perhaps, or extraordinary quantities of some particular vitamin. Nature seems to have been concerned only with this purpose.

For example, spinach gives us relatively tremendous quantities of Vitamin A, iron, and other minerals, considering its high water content and minute percentage of solids.

Nature is apparently willing that the body be forced to expend extra energy and work to dig out

85

these precious properties. Hence a catabolic food, while costing us a little fat and extra body energy, really gives a valuable return in the form of minerals and vitamins. Nature makes us work for the good things in food.

Study and consideration of the catabolic foods showed them to consist, chiefly, of those with a very high water content (such as cucumbers, 96 per cent water; cabbage, 94 per cent). The seventy-five really excellent catabolic foods are in the class called protective foods—those exceedingly rich in mineral and vitamin values, "healthful" foods.

Here was a stroke of luck. Imagine it: the very foods that contribute valuable vitamins and food minerals to the body turned out to be reducing foods.

A person twenty pounds overweight has 70,000 calories of stored fat. He could live for thirty-five days without any food—just water—and still do moderate work. Hence, it would seem decidedly beneficial for such a person to starve and use some of his burdening fat. But even a grossly overweight person must eat because food provides other necessary factors to life—vitamins, minerals, proteins, water, and so on. We must eat, even when reducing!

Additional inquiry into the catabolic foods showed not only mineral and vitamin values. Many of them were foods that provide an alkaline ash, very useful in offsetting the acid residue of fat destruction in the body. Furthermore, some of the catabolic foods were very rich in the food factors that have a favorable influence on the internal secretory glands.

The catabolic foods, as might be expected, were all very low in calorie value. When we figured up the daily calorie value of our L. C. diet, or its modification which became the reducing diet, the three pounds of food totalled only 600 calories on the average.

Here was another revolutionary turn. Many a dietitian vowed then that it was impossible to support life in an adult with only 600 calories per day. We knew that it was possible. For twenty years patients had lived for weeks and months on the L. C. diet and *thrived*. Patients had been *cured* of grievous disease by the L. C. diet, notwithstanding its low calorie value. *A 600 calorie per day reducing diet!* That's what the lady from Philadelphia led us to.

Just take a general view of the connotations of this discovery. First and foremost, here is a therapeutic diet which has made sick people well. Secondly, to lose fat efficiently on this diet, you have to eat, not starve yourself as some think. Furthermore, you have to consume large quantities of catabolic foods in order to lose weight rapidly. Eating large quantities of food to lose weight is something new for the fatty. But it is correct.

87

If the word *catabolic* is unwieldly or strange to you, call the catabolic foods "reducing" foods if you please. That is what they are. Or call them the "minus" foods, and weight-adding foods, the "plus" foods. In my daily tilting with Debble Fat, I keep a rummy score. I use points instead of calories, and I know that I have about 1800 points as my bank for the day.

A man of my size and activity needs about 1800 calories a day to live. If I, a lipophilic, eat more than 1800 calories' worth a day, I will store more fat. As I grow older and my metabolism rate diminishes, even 1800 calories will be too much.

Now if I should eat 1800 points of plus (fattening, anabolic) foods, I would be even-steven. Every time I eat a minus (thinning, catabolic) food, I am just that much ahead of Debble Fat for the day. Not only have I failed to add calories to my score, but I have actually trimmed some off.

See what a good game it is? Understand now why I don't have any worries about fat—why I have fun controlling my weight? It is far more interesting than bridge—and the stakes are higher.

Some days I eat six minus foods and only two plus ones. At other table sessions, I can't get out of eating too many plus foods. The next day I make up for it.

If I want a luscious, appealing plus food with plenty of calories as a main dish, I confound Debble Fat by compensating for my choice, somewhat, with minus foods in all the other menu rôles. He is a puzzled foe, Debble Fat, with this system.

You do have to know your foods with this system of weight control. You have to know something about any game you play—to win.

Let me tell you about some of these foods.

Note to readers versed in physiological chemistry: The heat and energy cost incurred in the metabolism of the catabolic foods must be considered distinct from the phenomena of specific dynamic action (S.D.A.).

The 6 per cent allowance made for increased metabolism due to food itself, as calculated in many standard diets, is excellent as far as it goes, but obviously the energy costs must vary with the type of food.

CHAPTER NINE

A Reducing Regime Is Evolved!

You MAY, if you wish, turn now to the calorie counter charts in the back of the book. I should prefer that you did not. Doggedly learning the calorie values of foods may not be such a great help to reducing as theory would have it. I think it would be much better to browse along for the next few chapters, and survey foods generally.

You know now that the secret of reducing is to eat the right kinds of foods. You know that proper reducing is not a question of starvation—of "cutting your meals in half." Best of all, you know that foods are not your enemies. You need not be afraid to eat, now. As a matter of fact, let us repeat our axiom: *You have to eat large amounts of catabolic foods to reduce.*

You may even agree that we can hope to cure the lipophilic of his difficulty by restoring catabolism and anabolism to a normal relationship. By our choice of foods we can surely condition the fat metabolism while its disturbances are still in a functional state.

In general, foods are your friends—always your friends, the best friends you have. They give you life and health. I don't suppose there is any food which does not contribute something of value to man's diet. But foods, like people, are individualistic; even one grain of wheat is different from another.

Foods have decided virtues and faults. We need some for one virtue; some for another. Some foods fit us; some foods fit the other fellow. Just as a businessman and a scientist, for their ultimate success and happiness, must select associates from different groups, so must we lipophilics choose our food intimates wisely.

The catabolic foods are overwhelmingly our best friends. Cultivate their companionship. You are going to be fashioned by the food company you keep.

The biggest handicap to reducing, according to most fat people, is the fact that many persons must eat in restaurants all of the time, and most of us have to eat in restaurants and friends' homes some of the time. As we go now to meet foods, let us consider them with the idea that we are going to use them in restaurants.

Salads: Here is Nature's gracious gift to us fatties. In the first place, salad ingredients are among the best and most pleasant foods with which to fight fat. Besides, they are the finest way in which to get the vitamins we need for health. The pill method of taking vitamins is all right as far as it goes, but it doesn't

91

go very far. There are important vitamins which have not yet been made available synthetically; there are more vitamins to be discovered in the future. Nature has put them all in foods.

Vitamins work together to produce special results, just as different notes, when played together, produce a musical chord. Food minerals also qualify and enhance the effect of the vitamins, a complex interplay still largely Nature's secret.

Chief among the vitamin values of salads is Vitamin C; its virtues are many. There is every reason to believe that the "four out of five" who have pyorrhea are largely so afflicted because they do not get enough Vitamin C. You see, if a person is sufficiently lacking in Vitamin C, he will develop scurvy. When Vitamin C is partially lacking in the daily diet, partial scurvy may develop.

Thanks to modern food distribution and knowledge, real scurvy is now quite a rarity. Once upon a time, however, especially on shipboard, it was a gruesome and deadly plague, altogether too frequent. Usually the first sign is bleeding gums. Many a ship's crew was thrown into terror and even mutiny when some hardy sailor would spy a blood stain on the bite of another sailor's biscuit and shout—"The scorby! The scorby is here!"

Vitamin C helps to prevent colds, catarrh, and other

such ailments. If we ate salads for no other reason in the world, they would be immensely worth while for their values in Vitamin C alone.

But salads are thinning. The best fat-blasting foods on the list are the salad vegetables such as lettuce, cabbage, and tomatoes. They are enemies, and respected ones, of Debble Fat.

The enjoyment of a salad depends upon the deftness and skill with which it is made. Salad making is an art—a high art. Salad vegetables must be crisp, chilled, and fresh as morning dew. Salad dressings are most important of all—just the right little dab of garlic, and for us you-know-whats, very little oil, if any. For nutritional reasons, we prefer lemon juice to vinegar. Besides being tastier, it is one of the richest of foods in Vitamin C.

If you will plan to have a salad served first at your main meal of the day, you have truly made a seven-league stride against Debble Fat. In the first place, that is the way a salad must be eaten if every nuance of taste and flavor is to be enjoyed and appreciated. And this question of flavor is important for us fatties, because we are entitled to enjoy every bit of food we eat to the nth degree. Goodness knows, there are enough tasty foods that we dare not eat.

The salad-first plan will stymie the bread-breaking habit. It wouldn't be so bad if we just broke the bread when we first sat down to the table. The trouble is, we not only break bread—we butter it and eat it in that gastronomical space of time between ordering and receiving a meal.

If I am extra hungry, and not at home where a salad is automatically served first, I always ask the waiter to bring some celery or sliced tomatoes while I study the menu. Then, while my table companions are eating bread and butter and debating the menu, I am slowly, deliberately—and thoroughly—enjoying celery, sliced tomatoes, radishes or some other fat-fighting relish.

Yes, the salad-first idea is a good one.

Soups: Soups are no problem to us lipophilics. Really, they are a decided help. There is always consommé, or some other clear soup available. If the soups on a particular menu happen to be the complicated sort, we should ask the waiter to strain them. Sometimes, of course, the menu is limited. There may be just one or two soups available—the rich, thick, creamy types at that. Beat a quick retreat, because a cream soup is very fattening.

Bouillons are certainly non-fattening, but they may be too salty, which does not help. Clear chicken soup and various clear broths are tasty and non-fattening, too. Be careful of broths, though. When rice or noodles swim temptingly in front of you, just leave them—they may cost you ten points (a ten-minute brisk run).

The julienne soups, canned or freshly made, are more thinning than bouillon because the vegetables have a minus value.

Chief opponents in the soup division are mushroom soup, which rates high in calories; bean soup (ten times as fattening as julienne); pea soup, a subtle sort of enemy; and tomato soup, which is a wolf in sheep's clothing because it is usually thickened with flour. Mulligatawny, clam chowder (the way it is usually made), oxtail and pepper pot soups can be trimmed down to our size by having them served clear.

Fatty soups, whether bought canned or prepared at home, can be compromised with in this way. Have your share of the soup placed in the refrigerator until the fat hardens a bit. Then the fat may be skimmed off and put back into the soup that goes to the rest of the family. Yours is served fat-free.

Tripper-Uppers: There are some tempting tripper-uppers among foods—take crackers, for example. They seem so harmless, so innocuous and so utterly innocent, especially those succulent little oyster crackers that seem to be mostly air. But they're not. They are made of flour, and while one or two little ones don't amount to much in calories, it never seems possible to stop at one or two, particularly when you are trying to outsmart Debble Fat by nibbling crackers to escape eating bread.

A half-cup of oyster crackers totals eighty-five calories. They may lose the day's match for you. Three soda crackers add up to fifty calories, which is too much. So it goes, down the whole list of crackers, for all of them—no matter what their trade names—still have calories. Beware!

While innocently listening to your neighbor's conversation, you can break a cracker into bits and put it into your soup. It is so easy, almost inevitable, to spread a bit of butter on the cracker, just a tiny little bit. Up goes the calorie count. The Swedish crisp breads of various types are, roughly, on a par with soda crackers in fattening value.

Breads: First we'll breathe a fervent prayer that all the numerous interests concerned with bread making will forbear their fury now. We fatties have a right to live, too.

I know as well as they do that the annual per capita consumption of breadstuffs has diminished most distressingly. I know that this hurts everybody in the industry, right down to the farmer.

But I also know that there are other food industries to engage in, and that an American farmer can raise something else besides wheat, rye, and corn on his soil. The major percentage of American farm lands is devoted to cereal raising, and there is such a glut of grains on the market that, first thing you know, our national wealth will be locked up in an ever-normal granary.

Orange growers have succeeded in creating a demand for their product, and the consumption of lettuce has jumped 1500 per cent within the last twenty years. With vastly improved methods of transportation and the miracle of quick-freezing, it should be no problem at all to build a greater public demand for the really excellent protective foods that grow in a garden.

I am of the personal opinion that with a few odd millions of dollars well spent each year to publicize the values of succulent garden vegetables, and to sell the American public on the idea of eating more of them, this demand could soon be created. It would be the healthful way to eat, and people generally like balanced eating after they have been shown the light.

If the American public ate a balanced diet—if it consumed only the milk, fruits, salad vegetables and greens that it should to maintain a *minimum* nutritional standard—farm income would be increased at least $3,000,000,000 per year. In addition we might need a little more farm land than is now in productive use.

With that introduction, we will consider breads. Let us have no misunderstanding. Bread is a very good food. Personally, I wish I were able to eat it with profit. But more fat doesn't profit me. A slice or two a day is all my competition with Debble Fat will permit.

Breads are fattening to lipophilics; no twisting of words will alter the situation. Bread is no longer the staff of life—not in this day and age when it is refined and there are hundreds of others foods readily available. And so, we who are fat have to consider bread as one of our A-1 opponents. But since bread is good to the taste, we naturally want some once in a while. So let's figure how best to fare with it.

Corn bread, delightful as it is, is a terrific handicap. One ordinary piece, about four inches square, counts up to nearly 275 calories all by itself. And how it does sop up butter! It's easy to run it up another 100 calories with just enough butter to make it tolerable. Last but not least, who of us, when eating corn bread, doesn't get the notion that a little syrup on it would be just yum-yum? Only a tablespoonful—only another seventy-five calories. There you are. We lose, double and redoubled.

There are only slight variations in the calorie values of ordinary breads. Strangely enough, whole wheat and rye breads are usually higher per slice than white varieties. But it's all a tempest in a teapot because the differences are so small, with the exception of gluten bread which has only two-thirds the caloric value of the others.

An ordinary slice of bread runs about sixty to sixty-five calories. That is not so much, and if you can confine yourself to one piece of bread at a meal, there is no harm done. But remember, the Damon and Pythias of foods are bread and butter. Personally, I find no pleasure in eating bread without butter. It is a glum, grim and wholly tasteless endeavor. Yet it may be by buttering bread that we give Debble Fat an advantage for the day.

For some reason, a great many people believe that rolls offer an escape from calories. They do not. Even those thin, papier-mâché types, of which restaurants seem to find unlimited quantities, are heavily calorific. Any and all of the various kinds will average around 150 calories each—double the caloric value of a piece of bread. And another catch is that, unless salted, they are utterly tasteless (nearer to the flavor of paper than any other food I know). They are so completely insipid that you have to load them with butter—so perhaps you had better ask for bread in place of rolls.

Home-made biscuits—ah, those delectable, delightful, fluffy temptations to obesity. A definite calorie value is difficult to assess because it will vary with the ingredients and the lightness or heaviness of the biscuit. Average figures for my cook's biscuits (a Southern cook of the first water) were as follows: twelve biscuits were made from a batch of dough containing 1200 calories' worth of ingredients. That averages 100 calories per not-too-big biscuit. Not bad, but biscuits were born to have butter on them, and they are forever flirting with jam (100 calories per tablespoon). Biscuits are a bother, no end. Ride a bicycle furiously one mile for every biscuit.

Cakes: Cakes are the Mata Hari's of foods, but since some are more so than others, it's worth while to figure out the least dangerous. After all, a man has to have a piece of cake once in a while.

Tenderly cutting the icing off a piece of cake and leaving it on your plate, or, better still, giving it to a tablemate who can take it, helps a little. With its contents of butter, sugar, cream, eggs, chocolate or whatnot, icing really has calories. But choosing a plain cake, if you have a choice, is best. The difference between a piece of chocolate layer cake and plain pound cake, for example, is worth considering: chocolate layer, 250 calories; pound cake, 180 calories.

When you select raisin pound cake, you win a couple of points because raisins replace some cake and are not as fattening. A standard piece of raisin cake counts 165 calories. On the other hand, a serving of walnut pound cake (one with just a skimpy amount of walnuts in it) counts 190 calories.

No, cakes are a siren lot, calorically speaking. The further we go into the matter, the more complicated it is likely to become. All told, angel food cake offers about the best out, as it has less flour and far more egg whites than most cakes. Yes, angel food or even a sponge cake—one small piece without icing—is a compromise of Fascist proportions.

Soda Fountain Seducers: A fatty at a soda fountain is a Daniel in the lion's den, especially if one of those super-skilled Dixie boys is behind the counter. You have undoubtedly run across members of this fraternity —debonair chaps who know just how to make a chocolate frosted to the queen's taste. The way they can sling calories into a dish or shaker is truly amazing. What's more, they have no compunctions about topping off the whole business with whipped cream.

Consider a malted milk:

malted milk	2 tablespoons	70 calories
chocolate syrup	3 ounces	325 calories
ice cream	1 gill (modest)	170 calories
milk	4 ounces	85 calories
	TOTAL	650 calories

Don't be misled into thinking this is an exceptionally high calorie rate, either. I have seen malted milks made much richer at many a drug store counter.

If you are at a soda fountain to tickle your taste
buds a bit, better order some plain ice cream. It is
toothsome, and a dandy food, as foods go, despite its
calories. But in considering ice creams, you get involved in some of the same problems that cakes present. When fruit is added, the calorie value is cut
down a trifle because the fruit takes up some room.
When nuts are added, the calorie value goes up because nuts are very fattening. Chocolate ice cream is
more fattening than plain ice cream.

When the fatty is tempted by a soda or a sundae, he
is really heading for trouble. As you should very well
know, ice cream syrups are mainly concentrated sugar,
and their calorie value will vary with the maker. Even
when you give them the benefit of every possible caloric doubt, you will have to figure that they average
about 500 calories to the half-cupful. And this amount
of strawberry or chocolate syrup is not as much as you
think. Just measure it and see. Such a portion of
syrup will dress a sundae immodestly and make a
thoroughly uninteresting ice cream soda.

No, soda fountain etiquette for the fatty should be
limited to orders of plain ice cream, phosphates, plain
sodas (strawberry, for example, without ice cream), or
some drink such as Coca-Cola, which contains only
sixty calories or so to the bottle. The really smart (with
a touch of Spartan) fatty calls for lemonade, orange

juice, milk, tomato juice or some other fat-escaping drink.

Tidbits: A census of the tidbits that modern ingenuity has devised to delight the palate would require practically a book in itself. These tantalizing traps for us lipophilics are laid everywhere, it seems. Most of us find cocktail crackers and potato chips, nuts of all sorts, popcorn, pretzels, pretzel sticks and various new and amazing tempters that came in with the repeal of prohibition, forever within reach. They are all fattening, drat 'em!

One average honest pretzel is worth about fifteen calories. Potato chips outrank pretzels, and nuts (although their fat content varies) are one almost as bad as another. If you want to get down to detail in the matter, peanuts (per ounce and *not* per nut, remember) are about the least fattening among ordinary varieties; pignolias come next, then cashews. Peanuts are perhaps only two-thirds as fattening as pecans. Walnuts, Brazil nuts, and almonds are about on a par and midway in caloric value between peanuts and pecans.

The best escape in tidbits is popcorn. Its intrinsic caloric value is less than any of the others, and besides, most of it is indigestible. The trouble with popcorn is that it requires butter and salt to be enjoyed. In fact the whole lot of tidbits are salty rogues, Debble Fat's allies from Lilliput.

Hors d'oeuvres: Now, of course, there are hors d'oeuvres and hors d'oeuvres. All of them are disarming because they are so petite and dainty looking, but some of them pack a hefty wallop in calorie value.

Consider the little cocktail frankfurters, for example, those tiny tempters-on-a-toothpick. They may seem "too small to count," but each of these tasty little squidgets averages seventy-five calories to the ounce, and it's easy to do away with an ounce of them. One taste simply calls for more.

The little pork sausages—they are really something. At 150 calories per ounce, porkies are rich in their own right, but now Debble Fat's agents have taken to wrapping a little piece of bacon around them. This means double trouble, for smoked bacon averages 130 calories per strip.

Other sausages, such as the liver and summer varieties, have simply tremendous calorie values. It's true that they are sliced thin and all that, but one slice never satisfied anyone. Summer sausage runs about 150 calories to the ounce, farm sausage 180, and bologna about 75, which makes the last-named our best bet in the sausage division.

Then there's that olive hors d'oeuvre. One green

olive, of ordinary size, means fifteen calories, which is bad enough in itself. Wound around with bacon and stuck on a toothpick, it would tempt a saint. There it is, decked out in another seventy-five calories.

Smoked fish is generally very fattening, although sturgeon and smoked salmon outrank the rest by far. Smoked halibut makes a hefty hors d'oeuvre, and unless your host has been kind enough to provide a bit of smoked haddock (which you rarely see), you had better reach for the celery instead of the fish.

Caviar is not so bad as you might think. A teaspoonful amounts to only twenty-five calories, and considering the fattening power of other hors d'oeuvres, that isn't much. The trouble is, there is never an abundance of caviar.

Other occupants of the canapé tray are usually made with creamy cheese, or else mayonnaise has played a rôle in the recipes. They are a hazardous lot for the fatty to survey even mentally, the hors d'oeuvres. The best thing to do is to fortify yourself with radishes and celery, if these have been provided. If not, bring your own, or set your will power to full speed ahead. Pardon me, your *won't* power!

Candy: Candies are legion and they are everywhere to be had. Even friends love to have candy bowls and boxes around for fatties to stumble on. When you consider that an ordinary piece of chocolate cream candy is worth 160 calories, you will get a rough idea of what we are up against. (Over half an ounce of fat to increase your curves unless you roller skate for an hour to use it up.) Bonbons and the cream fondants are almost as bad as chocolates.

No need to deny that candies are tempting. They are. Almost everyone has a sweet tooth, and ours is probably sharpened by our knowledge that sweets are forbidden. Chewing gum may help you to resist temptation, or, if you simply must have candy, buy the hard kinds. They last much longer, and you can wind up with a far better score than a couple of pieces of chocolate would give you.

Drinks: All alcoholic beverages, without exception, are fattening. There is no digestion cost; here is liquid fuel ready to be stored as fat.

Calorie values vary, of course, with the kind of drink. Beer of various types has a lower calorie count than wines and hard liquors (the lighter the beer, the fewer the calories). Since beer glasses differ in size, we had best give you the calorie values in cups: draft beer, 100 calories; bock beer, 135; ale, 150. Figure roughly an hour of badminton per glass of beer.

Wines can be assessed in wineglass portions (roughly three ounces): light, dry wines (French,

German, domestic, etc.), 75 calories. The sweeter or heavier the wine, the higher the calorie value: sherry, 140; muscatelle, 165; port, 165; dry champagne, 85; sweet champagne, 120.

Cordials are obviously fattening: anisette, 120 calories per *ounce*; benedictine, 112; kümmel, 75; crème de menthe, 105; maraschino, 112.

Among the hard liquors, the calorie values are approximately equal: bourbon, rye, and Irish whiskey, 85 calories to the ounce; gin, Scotch or rum, 75.

The calorie value of cocktails varies, of course, with the contents and the wishes of the mixer. I once went to the trouble of calculating the calorie value of some forty different common cocktails and, surprisingly enough, the general average was the same—about 80 calories per ounce (an hour of tennis).

The calorie count of alcoholic drinks is not the main handicap to the fat person; drinks stimulate the appetite and lessen the will to resist high-caloried foods. Or, if you want to put it the other way, drinks seem to give the fat person an unwarranted optimism which whispers, sirenlike, "Oh, what's the difference?"

Muscle Meats: It is absolutely necessary to life to have a few ounces of protein each day; for best health, it is essential to have some Class A proteins once in a while. (See *Glandular Meats*.)

107

Class B proteins are found in muscle meats—steaks, chops, roasts, and stewing meat. They are classed separately from glandular meats because, from a purely scientific standpoint, they are inferior builders of body tissue. They contain what are called Class B amino acids. And the amino acids are the little chemical bricks, so to speak, of which body cells are formed.

The first task we heavyweights have, of course, is to choose those meats which are intrinsically the least fattening. Then we must always cut away whatever fat may adhere to the serving.

When eating in restaurants, tell the waiter in clear tones that you like your meat lean. For home cooking --friend wife being willing—make special effort to buy lean pieces from the butcher. Muscle meats which have been hung have lower calorie value than those which are fresh. Besides, hanging adds immensely to their tenderness, digestibility, and flavor, so unless religious dietary laws prohibit their use, these should be chosen.

For the fatty, meats should be cooked and served in the simplest possible fashion. Where we usually get tripped up by Debble Fat is in the matter of garnishments, gravies, and fancy meat combinations. Since broiling renders meat of considerable fat, broiled meats are universally less fattening than meats cooked in any other form, including roasts. (Roasts are often heavily larded.)

Breaded meats run into dizzy caloric heights, not alone because of the breading but because the operation requires extra grease. Fried meats, of course, are absolutely taboo. Enough lard or butter will sometimes be sopped up in them to double or triple the original fattening value.

Meat pies are definitely on the suspect side. Not only do they have rich pastry coverings, but the pies themselves are liberally sprinkled with potatoes, and their succulent juices contain plenty of fat. Hashes, with their potatoes and various forms of fat, are also definitely *out*.

To summarize, we must ask for a lean slice of whatever roast is being served, or a lean, broiled steak or chop. If we choose chopped steak, we should request that any fat be laid aside before the meat is prepared for cooking.

The special gustatory appeal of a meat dish is often its sauce or gravy. What talent, art, and skill have been expended in fashioning these delights! They are most tempting—but they are for the four people out of five who are not fat, unless we can have a thin gravy made only of seasoned juices and a little water. Or our own cooks can put gravy into the refrigerator for its fat to congeal, and then serve us the delicious fat-free part which remains.

The garnishments—oh those tempting, ravishing

garnishments! Yorkshire pudding, potato croquettes, rissoles, timbales, and the countless other do-dads with charming names that chefs have been thinking up since civilization began. Pass them up, O fatty.

Poultry: Fowl is a muscle meat which ranks, as far as nutrition is concerned, with steaks, roasts, and chops. Duck waxes dangerous as a potential fattener, and goose must be left for our friends.

Although roasted fowl of any kind is mandatory in place of the more complicated concoctions of ingenious cooks, broiled chicken is our choice in young fowl. Fowl en casserole is far more fattening than roast fowl, while chicken croquettes, chicken patties, and such are super-highways to obesity.

Creamed poultry dishes are obviously fattening. Chicken à la king—even if you promise positively to pick out the chicken carefully and leave the rest—is taboo. It is from two to three times as fattening as a piece of chicken breast. And cooks just love to put creamed chicken into fattening crusts. It is even difficult to find a breast of guinea hen that has not been larded and nestled with a piece of ham on a slice of toast.

Stewed chicken is a safe venture, provided we pass by the luscious cream gravy, and leave noodles, dumplings and rice delights severely alone. Remember, too, that hominy, banana fritters and waffles are lieutenants in Debble Fat's army.

Fish: Fish is an excellent food, just loaded with food minerals from the sea. We can set aside heavy-handed custom, too, and serve fish on other days than Friday. Such a worthy food deserves to be eaten more frequently.

Since there are tremendous differences in calorie values, we must learn which kinds of fish are fattening and which are not. In general, fish dishes should be either baked or broiled. Fried and creamed fish are on the forbidden list.

As we know to our sorrow, fish offers unlimited scope to concoctors of sauces. Well, there's no use in setting our taste buds atwitter with vain recollections. Just remember that lemon juice is about as fine a flavoring agent as any fish could desire.

Lobster, oysters, shrimp, and clams are definitely the least fattening of protein foods. Besides, they are particularly rich in minerals—especially iodine, which spurs along metabolism. But these are best used as dinner appetizers or protein salads. After all, we do want some variety in those parts of our menus, and just as soon as these fish enter the entrée class, Debble Fat's agents seduce them.

What's the use of a broiled lobster without butter

sauce or mayonnaise? Lobster à la Newburg is three or four times more fattening than plain lobster. That is beyond all reason. We will eat lobster salad (made with chili sauce dressing).

Oysters give us a bit of a break. They are delightful baked with a little dab of chopped greens, a brisk brush of garlic and ever-so-few buttered cracker crumbs.

Let's save shrimp for salads or cocktails. If cooked, shrimp seems to demand to be creamed or curried—which takes it out of our class.

Glandular Meats: Glandular meats, such as brains, heart, kidney, liver, tripe, sweetbreads, lungs, spleen, and so on (tongue may be included), are man's finest sources of Class A protein. (Other sources are certain fish, eggs, milk, and soy beans among the vegetables.) These meats require parboiling, of course, to rid them of certain extractives, but they are excellent foods that are sadly snubbed by the American public. Primitive men and animals, existing by the rule of survival of the fittest, choose glandular meats in preference to muscle meats.

These are the chief meats which possess a real vitamin or mineral value. The curative quality of calf liver is but one example of their nutritional importance. That is the reason we will give them a frequent place on our menus. And as we go along, we will learn why the epicure smacks his lips over those meats which are too often thrown to dogs and cats, even as liver used to be.

It is true that some of these proteins are quite fattening, but we can dodge that effect by broiling them. A Sunday breakfast of broiled lamb kidney with eggs, for example, is not only tastier and far more valuable nutritionally, but is also considerably less fattening than ham, bacon, or country sausage with eggs would be.

Learn to like the glandular meats.

Eggs: Eggs, perhaps the most dependable source of protein known to early man, are among our trusted allies. Probably the most nearly perfect food nutritionally, they outrank milk (which is excellent, too, but far better advertised).

As long as eggs are going to be one of our protein mainstays, we should be acquainted with a number of tempting egg dishes—those, of course, which can be prepared in a suitable manner for lipophilics.

Boiled eggs are best from the calorie viewpoint. They may be boiled to any degree we desire, although we might ask that they *not* be cooked in furiously boiling water (slow-cooked eggs are always more digestible). Baked eggs that have escaped fattening ad-

113

ditions are all right, but fried eggs have a calorie value two or three times higher than that of their simple boiled cohorts.

Eggs scrambled slowly and lightly in a pan dabbed with just enough butter to prevent sticking are friends. We can also stave off Debble Fat with a plain omelette. But the cook who wields a mighty butter or grease spoon can add so much fat to scrambled eggs that their calorie value may be doubled, tripled or quadrupled. And we take a real setback with fancy omelettes, especially creamed ones.

For you who miss the friendliness of bacon or ham with eggs, we recommend this tasty substitute: soak the salt out of a bit of chipped beef, pan-broil lightly, and serve just as you would its more pound-adding predecessors.

Dairy Products: The dairy products include an assortment of food friends that rate aces high. Here are man's most dependable sources of food calcium, from which bones and tissues are knit and teeth built. Dairy foods should comprise a sizable portion of man's meals, and account for a generous slice of his food dollar.

We lipophilics have to watch our way, though, in dairyland. After all, we don't need much food fat, and as it is present to some degree in most substances, we get essential lipoids and fatty acids in tidbits here and there.

Two of our best choices are skim milk and butter-milk, from which most of the calorie-rich cream has been removed. We have to watch our P's and Q's with cream. If we must add something to a cereal or bever-age, let's choose light cream—or, even better, whole milk. Using cream instead of milk is largely a matter of habit and custom. We can soon learn to enjoy the less fattening liquid, even in coffee or tea.

Whipped cream is a lily-white, pure, clinging-vine type of seducer among Debble Fat's minions. Some cooks apparently believe it just has to be served with every dessert and some salads. Let them have their way, but resolutely peel off the whipped cream. If your will power is good, leave it on your plate. If not, either pass it on to somebody who looks hungry, or pour salt and pepper on it. That will discourage you from forming *anschluss* with it or putting it in your coffee. Just a dab of whipped cream, 70 calories, calls for fifteen minutes of vigorous work.

Butter is one of the finest of foods, and particularly valuable for its Vitamin A content. In addition, it has special lipoids and fatty acids which rank with the A-1 amino acids as food factors necessary to life.

While we are following the strict reducing diet, we can afford to let butter go by because the seven-day diet is more than rich in Vitamin A foods. But if we are just coasting along and watching ourselves carefully, we can use modest amounts of butter, well aware that it is fattening, but equally sure that it is one of the best foods. Judgment—that is all we need.

The over-buttering of vegetables practiced so ardently by many cooks is a snare for the fatty. It is superseded, as a Debble Fat plot, only by the sugaring of every conceivable vegetable (mainly in the Eastern states).

Vegetables should be dressed with their own pot liquors and a dab of seasoning.

Cheese is a far better protein than the muscle meats. It is worth more, in essential amino acid value, than any steak, chop or roast you ever ate. To collect such extra food dividends, we can have a cheese soufflé, or a bowl of pot cheese, more than occasionally for a vegetarian lunch or dinner.

Take a good look at the fattening values in our calorie counter, and choose the lower-caloried cheeses. Then give this food the nutritional respect it deserves; eat it as the meal's main protein, not just a tacked-on afterthought. Tough, hardy desert Arabs live, love and fight on a bowl of cheese and some dates.

Vegetables: Vegetables, together with fruits, are, all told, our richest source of vitamins and minerals. We fatties can comfort ourselves by remembering that the skinnies and normals should eat a lot of vegetables, too, probably twice or three times as much as the average person does. They will have their nutritional troubles if they don't. So there is some consolation in our having to eat vegetables for double-chinned reasons. We will probably be healthier, after a given number of years, than our spinach-scorning confrères who are not lipophilic.

Not the least amazing feature of vegetables is their variety and abundance. Despite this, the average housewife or chef has a limited list of perhaps eight vegetable acquaintances. There are twenty or thirty tasty members of the plant kingdom which many cooks simply don't know exist.

Frequently people shudder at the mere mention of vegetables. I don't blame them—they have probably never tasted well-cooked ones. Culinary atrocities are certainly committed daily in thousands of homes when such foods as greens, cabbage, and spinach are prepared for dinner (like boiled blotters). Yet vegetables can be prepared in such delicious fashions; it is only that few of us know how. The man who remarked that God made foods and the devil made cooks must have been thinking of these much-maligned gifts of Mother Nature—vegetables.

The situation is doubly regrettable because the

biological function of vegetables is to supply us with vital vitamins and minerals, and improper cooking can destroy some or all of the vitamin value. Bad cooking wastes more than half the mineral value of vegetables, too. When nutrition scientists begin to rewrite our cookbooks, chapters on vegetables will bear the brunt of revision.

We feel sorry for those people who have religiously eaten vegetables for health purposes only to find after a time that they were still sick. They have a right to say that vegetables did them no good. They found out by experience. But it was the cooking method—not the carrots or beets—which failed. Vegetables cooked with an eye to their mineral and vitamin preservation would probably have accomplished the job in view. The highest art in food preparation, we believe, lies in vegetable cookery. Certainly that is where the science of cooking resides.

Brightly burnished microscopes in a nutrition laboratory, voluminous diet books on library shelves, will never cure Weary Wilhelminas of pernicious anemia. Neither will the marvelous knowledge lodged in a doctor's brains. *Eating calf liver will.*

It is what you *eat* that will cure you or hurt you, dietetically. So the science of nutrition rests ultimately upon the shoulders of the housewife, the homemaker, and the cook.

Education is the key!

Naturally the "best" vegetable is the one in season —a vegetable fully ripened, grown in good soil and brought to the kitchen as soon as possible. It should be quick-cooked, and its juices and pot liquors served with it. The goal to strive for is preservation of body. When vegetables are cooked to the mushy stage, ill has been done.

Remember, too, that most vegetables were meant to be mixed with each other. Nature provides some with tart or sharp tastes and others that are absolutely bland. Once their fine, delicate flavors have been preserved with quick and expert cooking, the art of preparation is encompassed by learning which vegetables to use with others. The judicious use of a little onion, tomato, mint, parsley or other flavoring agent will also be of considerable help. String beans may call for a little dab of chopped onion; spinach can be mixed with a few lettuce leaves; white turnips may be diced and cooked with their own chopped leaves. The Chinese, with their ancient civilization, have developed this technique of vegetable combination to the nth degree.

Just study the list of vegetables and see how uniformly low their calorie values are. Not that almost every vegetable has a lower value cooked than when raw. Pay special attention to the division marked "best eaten cooked" and "best eaten raw" because nutritional balance demands that some raw vegetables or foods be eaten every day.

Furthermore, some of the garden vegetables, rarely served cooked in the average American home, are epicurean delights. For example, consider celery, stewed gently and quickly in a bit of skim milk, then flavored with its own leaves and a touch of onion. Radishes are equally tasty when prepared in this fashion. A few radish leaves make a tasteful addition to salads, too.

Cucumbers, Chinese cabbage, and celery cabbage leaves can be cooked in a jiffy and are delicious.

Mixed greens (*fines herbes* is their seventy-five cent name) are usually a combination of the invaluable leaves thrown away by most housewives. Thus, beet and turnip greens may be added to the outer leaves of lettuce or cabbage. Such dishes are the food iron mines of Dame Nature.

And all these strangers to the average American cook are low-caloried, catabolic gifts to the fatty, besides being economic royalists in the vitamin world.

Fruits: Fruits, which are probably the masterpieces among protective foods, have been put by Nature into such attractive packages that we are tempted to eat them raw, which is best. There are a few which can sustain life all by themselves, and as a whole they are our main source of Vitamin C. In our war against

Debble Fat, we count fruits the flying cavalry, or—to be more modern—the air service.

Fruits can make up a breakfast for us, and a dandy one at that. They provide an escape for the fatty who is not satisfied by a snack and a cup of coffee for that meal.

Fruits can also solve the dessert problem, and believe me, it is a weighty one. Most people with any sort of an appetite want a sweet at the end of a meal, and desserts are apt to be a pitfall to fatties until they learn to use fruits for that purpose. A fruit cup dessert is comforting, satiating, yet not calorically dangerous.

Of course some fruits are exceedingly rich in sugar. We will leave them for other people. But the handsome varieties we *can* eat, we should enjoy chilled, stewed, fresh, or in fruit cups of endless combinations.

Fruits help solve the problem of hors d'oeuvres and meal beginnings, too. A half-grapefruit, a slice of melon, or a fruit juice cocktail makes a perfectly delicious appetizer. For those very few people who just "can't stand" vegetables of any kind, fruits are perfect vegetable substitutes. Although it is not a custom with us and may seem strange to conventional eaters, fruit dishes may be served instead of vegetable dishes. Prunes with heavy meat dishes help. Pineapple or apples help "cut" rich meats. Rhubarb and stewed fruits of various kinds may serve as vegetable side dishes—they lend variety, too. As a matter of fact, some of the foods which we call vegetables, such as tomatoes, are really fruits.

Nibblers are offered an escape by fruits. An apple or an orange can always be selected in place of some fattening tidbit between meals, or when time hangs heavy on our hands.

Housewives, especially young brides, are prone to become nibblers and snack eaters. Just 100 unneeded calories a day, a cocktail, a snibble of candy, a cookie or a whatnot, worth identical calories when stored as fat, equal ten pounds a year. Nibble some fruit if you must.

Nibblers can't see a movie without a nickel's worth of candy (1000 calories?). Ball games, shopping tours —in fact, all expeditions—are punctuated by nibbles. A Sunday drive in the car equals one hot dog, assorted popcorn and sweetmeats, ice cream cones and what have you—enough calories to drive the car. It's a bad habit—nibbling.

I, personally, am a congenital refrigerator raider. This habit I came by honestly from my father and mother. Well, icebox raiding is one of the few joys that most men can still indulge in. So far neither dictatorship nor emergency legislation has interfered with it.

But obviously, undisciplined raiding can run a fatty

into trouble. There is usually cheese or left-over meat to tempt one. Both are doubly bad because they invite just a bit of bread and butter to make a sandwich.

It is all solved when there is fruit in the icebox, and even the humblest mortal can manage to have this around. I have centered on apples, and now have the habit of eating one every night so firmly ingrained that nothing else would tempt me and certainly not satisfy me. I make a ceremony out of it—it is worth one. The apple is cool and firm. I peel, quarter, and munch it philosophically.

I have to battle for the privilege, in a mild way, with my old Scotty and Tough Tim, a Kerry blue. They are wise to the bedtime snack. They know it is going to happen every night and they are ready. My share has been cut to three-quarters of an apple because the dogs can detect the faint sound of an apple being peeled at least three rooms away. They run to sit at my side with respectful attention and imploring eyes. But do you think those dogs will eat an apple with peeling on it? Not on your life, yet I remember the day when they were happy with a core!

Yes, fruits are one of the best allies we fatties have.

CHAPTER TEN

Our Diet Makes Its Debut

THE WAR of 1914 brought to light such important knowledge in scientific nutrition that research in dietetics surged forward by leaps and bounds. The baby science of nutrition was now in its swaddling clothes. Father was deeply gratified; he began to formulate new plans.

We had always realized that operating a sanitarium to demonstrate the importance of diet was far from ideal. Patients who come to a sanitarium are usually at the tag end of a disease. Often the best that can be done is to mitigate their symptoms and give them a little further breath of life, which, of course, is not the ultimate function of diet.

The greatest value of nutrition lies in the prevention of disease, in the building of super-health, and in the prolongation of years of life. Obviously, the most useful and needed service that a practicing nutritionist could render would be to teach people how to eat to have health, to instill the importance of nutrition into mothers, so that they could have better babies and feed their children for optimum health.

By 1922, my father was definitely convinced that it was time to bring the newer knowledge of nutrition directly to the public. This meant teaching homemakers reform in cooking methods and revolutionary changes in the customary menu planning. Intelligent eating demands an entire redistribution of foods in the diet of the average person, with far more vegetables and fruits and less of starches and proteins.

Father began to prepare for the new work. He placed the Sanitarium property on the market for sale. Then an accident intervened, which later caused his death.

Just how our new plans would have evolved had Henry Lindlahr lived longer, only Providence knows. To teach nutrition to the public can be accomplished in many ways. That our plans would find ultimate fulfilment by what in those days was a squawking gadget called the radio was inconceivable. Such, however, was Fate's decree.

By chance, in the summer of 1929, I had the opportunity to deliver some diet talks over the radio. The listeners' response truly amazed me. People *were* interested! There are no words to describe my feelings when I realized that here was the way to teach nutrition. From that moment on, the microphone became my very life.

The literally stupendous portent of broadcasting as a medium for disseminating what I hold to be priceless knowledge was augmented by the thrill and satisfaction of "meeting" thousands of nice people interested in the same ideas that I am. I love it—I always shall.

Mrs. Jones' problem with Papa Jones who will have no "truck with bunny food," Mrs. Smith's gain of three pounds in one week—such and a hundred other adventures fill every day. The twaddle of critics, "It's all so irregular" (and worse) makes life more interesting. It is satisfying, worth while. I am still afraid sometimes that I will wake up to find it all a dream.

Our radio program has always been an informal one, in fact very informal. We hobnob with the radio listeners, read their letters, opinions and comments, and try to mold the broadcasts according to the suggestions and desires of the listeners. The constant theme, of course, is nutrition.

Many, many listeners wanted the text of the broadcasts in black and white. We began the *Journal of Living,* the first lay nutrition journal, I believe. It has prospered.

Naturally, questions on reducing and the problem

of what to eat and what not to eat in obesity were of paramount interest to listeners. From 1929 to 1935 we sent out hundreds of copies of our reducing diet, embodying the catabolic principles, to interested listeners. The results were uniformly excellent.

Here the 600-calorie diet showed its worth in the crucible of clinical tests. Stop to consider that in medical literature and practice prior to 1938, it was held:

1. *That a reducing diet of 1500 calories a day was about the greatest calorie restriction permissible.*

2. *That it was not safe to lose more than two or three pounds a month.*

3. *That any reduction of weight at the rate of a pound a day must be deadly and dangerous.*

I thought differently, of course, but established opinions about diet change slowly, even in scientific circles.

Then something happened. Early in July 1935, a group of radio listeners suggested that we actually broadcast a reducing diet and give the menus day by day in detail. I jumped at the idea. If a considerable number of the audience would go on the diet, follow it faithfully, and then report, we would really accumulate irrefutable evidence and the not-to-be-denied attention value of the spectacular. So, we agreed a few

127

weeks later, the audience and I, that we would try a test reducing diet if a thousand listeners would promise to follow.

We added that if the test were satisfactory from the audience viewpoint—if it actually helped procrastinating, weak-willed overweights to undertake a "mass" reducing effort—we would follow the test with a reducing party for all of the audience who wished to take off weight in good company.

A few weeks later we began the test diet. About 1100 people started out. By the time the *Journal of Living* went to press, we had received 438 reports. Within a month, 936 had reported—the average weight loss on the test party had been one pound a day for ten days.

The test had further demonstrated the worth of the catabolic diet. I tightened up the diet, shortened the time to seven days, and made ready for our first radio reducing party. In April 1936 we had the party and 26,000 listeners participated! This time we sent out mimeographed notes containing the diet menus in detail. The average loss of weight was eight pounds in seven days (all cases).

Following the "big" party, the reducing diet was printed in formal style. One of the primary principles in the diet was decidedly conducive to furthering the use of one of my sponsor's products. The sponsor helped considerably in obtaining a distribution of the diet notes in New York and Philadelphia.

The sale of the notes was phenomenal. An edition of 200,000 copies was exhausted within a year. Additional printings were made. By the Fall of 1938, close to a half million copies had been sold. Evidently, considerable numbers of people, in this wide land of ours, were using the Lindlahr reducing diet.

Concurrently with this widespread public reception of the catabolic reducing diet, medical literature pertaining to obesity and reducing underwent considerable change. Finally, in the *Journal of the American Medical Association* (December 10, 1938), a most amazing case was reported in detail. It was the history of a woman who had reduced from 395 to 156 pounds in twenty months.

1. The patient had been kept on a 600-calorie diet —a diet similar to ours.

2. The basic conclusion drawn from the study was: "There is no limit to the extent to which excess weight may be removed by low-calorie diets, provided they contain the necessary proteins, minerals, and vitamins."

The medical concept of the dietary treatment of obesity was sharply revised. Thus a principle went into practice! Thus a 600-calorie diet was "approved."

129

Now perhaps a dip into the transcribed notes of our broadcasts during the reducing party, and excerpts from some of the letters written by participants, will give some of you hesitating, procrastinating mortals with nebulous fears of what might happen if you were to follow our reducing diet, an actual view of what really happens.

On April 27 we began the diet. As we gave the daily menus over the air that week and encouraged listeners to stick to their guns, hundreds of people who went on the diet were kind enough to phone, write, or even telegraph their progress. What a hectic week that was, the reducing party!

Let us look now at bits of some of the letters broadcast. See how people fare on our diet. It is revealing.

Fifth Day of the Diet (May 1)

Mrs. R.H.G., Homesburg, Pa.: I am on your list of reducers. I weighed 192 on Monday (such a surprise when I got on the scales). I weighed 190 on Tuesday, and boy, was I feeling good? I housecleaned for four hours, then went to the movies.

I haven't eaten a piece of bread or a spoonful of sugar. And I've pulled in my girdle about three inches. . . .

I tried to interest my two daughters-in-law—nothing doing. They say diets are dangerous, but I'll show them. . . . Puffiness out of my ankles and shin bones . . . rediscovering the buoyancy of health, head clear as a crystal.

I vowed I was going to get my girlish figure back, and I'll show some certain snooty young ladies that they don't know it all, not by a jugful."

From a night nurse in Brooklyn: Well, I, for one, feel it's a real duty to tell you the results of the present reducing diet. Am I losing? Well, I certainly am. I'm one of the great army of fat night nurses. . . . I have to have a bite with the family and eat at home, too. Have to eat meals at night while on duty because I'm on the go then. I have a little bit of toast and coffee in the morning. Result: six or seven meals in twenty-four hours.

Does a night nurse get fat? You know she does! I am perfectly satisfied with the reducing meals and the discipline. No need to tell you I'm feeling 100 per cent fit. I can hardly eat all the food given in a meal and the feeling of satiety stays with me until the next one. I like this diet better than your test diet of last year.

Sixth Day of the Diet (May 2)

From a lady in New York City: I wish to report a loss of four pounds on the fourth day. Isn't that grand? I'm the lady who inquired how I could go on the diet when so many vegetables were listed, and I couldn't chew because of lack of teeth. A friend of mine suggested that I grind the vegetables. That's just what I'm doing, and here I am, losing at the rate of a pound a day. I'm going to take off thirty pounds before I get through.

A letter from a gentleman: Foolishly or otherwise, I allowed my wife to cajole me into going on your diet. She

131

got in her insidious work when I had just finished one of my favorite meals. I had never eaten carrots, spinach, squash, or most of your non-fattening vegetables in my life. I utterly despised them so you can imagine what a time I am having with your meals. It's tough trying to force them down.

And the raw salads—boy, they are terrible. But I ate according to prescription except for last night, when I took a flop. I had three beers and a pretzel. This morning I arose full of remorse, and right back on the diet I went. I weigh only 165 but am too fat for my height. I should get down to 140. I have lost a couple of pounds but I am afraid to go near a scale.

Another letter from a gentleman in New York City: On April 27, I weighed 231 pounds. Waistline forty inches, calf eighteen, thigh twenty-seven, hip girth forty-five, height six feet one, age 43. On May 2, I weighed 224 pounds, waist thirty-eight and one-half inches, calf seventeen, thigh thirty-five, hips forty-four. I lost exactly eight pounds.

I possess a heavy, bony structure, and I want to add, for I am associated with well-rated medical men, that your diet is unquestionably the best organized, most scientific of any I have seen.

A lady in Philadelphia: Lost six and one-half pounds from Monday until Friday. . . . As I wrote you previously, I have diabetes. During the five days, my blood sugar dropped from 220 to 137½. I was so surprised that I asked my doctor if that were possible. He said of course it was, and that I was doing fine.

The Following Monday

From Philadelphia: I am 50 years old, five feet two, and weighed 259. Began the diet April 27 without much hope, as I had been told that it was impossible for me to reduce. Tuesday morning, I hadn't lost an ounce, but I can figure why now, because my elimination was thrown off balance.

Wednesday, I almost popped off the scales from surprise, because I had registered a three-pound loss. I couldn't believe it. Happy? No words to describe it! By Thursday, I had lost five pounds. I had been in the habit of drinking nine to twelve cups of coffee and glasses of water a day. I imagine I was sometimes waterlogged.

By Saturday I had lost nine pounds. I told my butcher; he wouldn't believe me. And now, Monday morning, after a net loss of twelve and one-half pounds, I feel splendid and have a big day's work mapped out.

There you are, good reader. That's a gnat's eye view of the beginning days of the diet.

The final survey of that week's adventure showed that the catabolic diet, when used in thousands of cases, worked—really worked—with the accuracy of the law of averages.

Eight Pounds in Seven Days: Here unquestionably was the wave in the surge of human affairs that washed away the fear of low-calorie diets! Here was begun an accumulation of evidence and experience

that has changed the present-day scientific reducing
diets to a 600-calorie basis.

Here a groundwork was laid for the revolutionary
present-day medical principle—"There is no limit to
the extent to which excess weight may be removed. . . ."

CHAPTER ELEVEN

Pilgrims' Progress in Reducing

THE AFTERMATH of our radio reducing party brought thousands upon thousands of letters. Out of them we selected some 9,000 for our permanent files and these letters, I am sure, contain an unexampled store of information about weight control. Of course countless questions were asked but even more were answered, and we were given precious information which was detailed entirely in terms of human experience.

Here was knowledge that could scarcely be supplied from abstract reasoning or theory or even gained in searching laboratory experiment. Perhaps if we browse about among these letters for a few pages, it may prove interesting. Some of the thoughts we glean may be repetitious. But then again we may gainfully augment what information we have already gathered.

If we learned nothing else, we learned that the exaggerated taste for fattening foods, which is a pitfall for so many lipophilics, is usually nothing more or less than a fault born purely of habit. It would be interesting to know just what percentage of fat people are overweight because they eat too much sugar, starch, or fat. Our letters tend to show that it is the starchy foods that seem to be the most usual hazard for the overweight.

In fact, quite often our overweight listeners vowed that they just didn't like fat and couldn't eat it. But they would confess a tremendous liking for starches and sweets. Certainly it was a definite trait among our fatties and I wonder if the tendency isn't born of mankind's dim experience of the past.

It is very difficult in this day of great plenty in foodstuffs to realize that only a few generations ago practically all mankind lived in fear of starvation and famine. Railroads, motorcars, steamboats have enabled us to shift foods from one part of the world to another and surpluses from here to there.

Before improved transportation methods, if there were a drought, pestilence, or crop failure in some part of the world, the evil could not be alleviated, for food could not be moved to the stricken region quickly enough. So for thousands and thousands of years, most of mankind was unused to plenty, and perhaps it thus became ingrained in man to eat too much when there was enough food around.

Now if there is any truth in this idea, if it serves as an excuse for the human habit of eating too much, then perhaps we can reason that the inordinate desire of many people for too much starchy food is just a carry-over from former times.

Until perhaps the year 1800, in most parts of the world cereals were the mainstay of the human diet. Throughout Europe, rye bread was the chief food. Meat was a rarity. Cattle were used for ploughing and other farm work. They were much too valuable to be used for food until they were so old that they could not work.

Farm methods were crude and inefficient. Perhaps ten bushels of grain was a good yield for an acre of land in a year. With not enough grain to feed the populace, it is not surprising that farm animals were not raised for food. The gardening of common greens and vegetables is a comparatively new advance. This custom did not appear in England until about the time of Henry VIII.

Such foods as cabbages, turnips, radishes, and onions were used in olden times only as medicinal herbs. Perhaps the use of potatoes, which were brought from South America in the middle of 1500's and which came into common use in Western countries 100 or 150 years later, was the revolutionary change that gave mankind a more liberal diet.

Be that all as it may, when the human species for thousands of years has subsisted upon cereals or, in other words, a preponderantly starch diet, it is not easy to pry the "taste" loose. But it can be done, and proof of this fact to my mind was the most important lesson that I gleaned from our post-reducing-party letters.

When one-time fatties wrote, as they did by the hundreds, that they had learned to like the non-fattening fruits and vegetables and that it was no longer a problem for them to pass by starches and sweets, great progress had been made.

When a person eats a starchy food, some of it is very quickly converted into sugar—which in turn sends up the blood sugar. The blood sugar rise gives the person a lift not unlike that of alcohol. Depending upon or craving this stimulus or lift can be a habit and sometimes a vicious one, an appetite which is at least no help to the fatty—for the fat which is made from starches is a "hard fat" more difficult to break down than some others.

In this same vein of thought, we learned again the salutary lesson that there is a tremendous difference between appetite and hunger. Hunger is comparatively easy to appease; appetite is not. Appetite will remain with a person long after hunger has been satiated. How easy it is to dive into that rich, luscious dessert even though you are full to the bursting point of meat and other dishes of the table!

But we found, too, that appetite, at least an exaggerated appetite, for foods can be squelched. Our custom of eating a salad first or a goodly portion or two of the non-fattening fruits or vegetables before we look with favor upon the breads or other fattening foods is the best prophylactic against appetite indulgence.

We learned that following the catabolic system of eating over a reasonable period of time often engineered that most desirable of accomplishments—the destruction of fat where it most needs to be destroyed. In freak diet reducing systems, or where exercise is depended upon, very often the fat person will lose fat mainly in the skin and neck, becomes drawn and haggard looking, but still exhibits the fat paunch, the "spare tire." I could give you deep and complicated reasons for this phenomenon. It has to do with the different types of fat which accumulate in different parts of the body.

The human body maintains fat depots. The skin is one. So is the lower abdomen and that section in the midriff which doctors call the omentum. The fat stored in the depots is apt to be of a little different composition from that in other parts of the body and more difficult to break up by ordinary body metabolic processes.

The introduction of a goodly percentage of foods in the diet which stir up and stimulate the catabolic processes so heightens the destruction of fat that even

139

the tougher kinds are blown up. The thyroid and other glands are stimulated to greater activity by the catabolic diet. At any rate, hundreds and hundreds of our listeners who followed the reducing diet and later chose catabolic foods more liberally reported that the spare tire, the extra chins, or the alderman had obligingly disappeared.

We learned that the curve of fat destruction paralleled in intensity, roughly, those periods of life when fat is ordinarily less likely to accumulate. Briefly, it is a bit more difficult to reduce an infant than it is a child. People in their 20's, 30's and 40's reduce more easily than those in their 50's and 60's, but those in their 70's and on, reduce the easiest of all.

It is amazing how closely these observations tally in so-called fat storage cycles in human life. Physiologists tell us that it is normal for babies to be fat, children to be lean, young adults to be even leaner. It seems average for people in their 50's and 60's to be fatter, and it is normal and natural to grow thin in old age.

We also tried to do an interesting bit of detective work, but doing it by mail was clumsy and unsatisfactory. Some day someone will pursue the trail and discover some interesting facts. Here is the thought.

You undoubtedly appreciate by now that there are special metabolic processes for sugar, fat, and starch, each very intricate. That is not even half of it. There are special considerations for different kinds of sugar and fat, and obesity problems to be solved in the study of any of these problems.

For example, different fats are absorbed by the body in greater or less degree, more slowly or more rapidly as the case may be. The fat of olive oil is absorbed quicker than the fat of butter. In animals the type of fat fed will be the type of fat found in their tissues. A similar process goes on in man. The fat of a corn-fed hog is different from that of a slops-fed hog. Hogs fed peanuts or soy beans have particular fats differently flavored, differently composed.

It is quite possible to understand why some people gain weight more rapidly than others, by examining the *type* of fatty foods or sugars and starches they like to eat. Various sugars are used by the body more readily than others, or made into fat more easily.

It gets down to pretty fine points, intensely interesting, and promises that some day we can have reducing diets much more liberal in fats and starches than our catabolic diet, for example. But first we will have to learn a lot more about food chemistry.

You might remember, though, that the *fruit sugars* so liberally supplied in our diet have a low absorption rate, and are much better for the fatty than cane sugar or other types.

Another mystery we hoped to solve was why an in-

dividual sometimes exhibits a much more rapid conversion of starches into fats than usual. In other words,
sometimes it is very much easier to put on *fat* than at
other times—sometimes one has to be *very* careful about
calories; at other times one can get away with a lot. We
have some good clues but not the answer.

Checking 500 men of all ages and sizes who went
on the reducing diet against 500 women who reported
concurrently, we found that men lose faster than
women or, to be more exact, that they lose more weight
by a few ounces, almost half a pound, than women do
in the same seven days.

This may be readily explained by the fact that the
metabolism rate of men is on the average higher than
that of women. Particularly there is a very great difference in the special starch and sugar metabolism of the
sexes. This difference is based on the needs of child
bearing and is arranged by the interaction of the sex,
adrenal, and pituitary glands. In practice, it means
that a woman is more apt to make starches and sugars
into fat, more apt to gain weight, and somewhat more
difficult to reduce.

All in all, by far the greatest gains in health, well
being, and general fitness were made by our overweight
friends who were beyond the age of 50. To some extent
this might be due to the fact that listeners beyond that
age are more interested in health and much more likely

to follow directions closely—more determined to reduce. More significantly, however, those beyond 50 are likely to have rheumatism, high blood pressure, gall bladder trouble, and the degenerative diseases.

Naturally their dividends from reducing would be far greater than those of people who are not afflicted. The connection between overweight and some of the degenerative diseases is so close that reducing becomes an essential part of the alleviation of these ailments. So we are not surprised at the volume of reducers who report that high blood pressure went down from ten to fifty points, or that their blood sugar diminished 10, 20, 50, or even 100 per cent.

Elsewhere we have mentioned that excess pounds become much more burdensome with advancing years —symptom producing—and the aging body is correspondingly grateful for loss of weight.

I took the trouble to write some hundreds of our regular listeners who reported that they had kept their weight loss and not allowed themselves to gain weight again, to ask them why. Did they keep their pounds down because of appearance, because they looked better, or because they had some symptom which they wanted to control? What was the impelling reason?

When we set aside those answers which gave a serious health motive such as the control of blood pressure or the attempt to fight diabetes, a great, great majority reported that they held their weight down because they felt better when they were not too fat.

This could hardly be called a scientific reason but it is obviously a practical and impelling one. Fat accumulates upon most of us so insidiously that we little realize the burden it is until we have had a dramatic chance to go along without it for a while. When we find how much better we feel with ten pounds off, how much more pep we have, how much greater our energies, our capacities, and enjoyment of living, then only do we appreciate the full value of being normal in weight.

Taking the gain of feeling better in a more specific sense, we found that those ladies who found an increase of weight coincident with the change of life felt the "most better," if we may be allowed to distort the king's English so flagrantly. We noted also that the fat which accumulates at this period of life seemed to be a little more easily demolished than ordinary fat accumulation.

Twenty-five women in the New York, New Jersey, and Philadelphia areas who were more than thirty-five pounds overweight and definitely in the change of life reduced an average of $9\frac{3}{25}$ pounds on the seven-day diet, according to their letters.

We found, as might be expected, that most of the young men and women in their early 20's were reducing only for the sake of appearance. They were usually content to take off five, six, or ten pounds. They were inclined to allow fat to accumulate once more—then the diet was repeated. On the other hand, youngish actors and actresses and, strangely enough, young matrons who had taken on too much weight after the babies came, were very diligent about keeping the pounds off, once they had reduced.

Suspicions gleaned from the letters were many, but among them were these—that the Lady Stayabeds who liked to have their breakfasts in bed and who had the leisure time to indulge the idea, were the ones who were most likely to find fault with the diet, to give it up, or to complain that they got nowhere with it.

Surprisingly many people have no idea that cocktails, wine, or other alcoholic drinks add calories to the diet.

The typical housewife, homemaker, and good mother is very often a slave to the snack habit. Her great difficulty is that she has a little spot of tea or coffee here and there or she attends too many socials, bridge parties, or club meetings that give her an extra meal during the day. She nibbles too much.

Bread eating seems to be the chief hazard of many overweight men—lots of bread and butter. Big lunches seem to be the businessman's bane—that and the excuse that he is going to take off the extra pounds with exercise some time or another.

It was surprising and comforting to note the really tremendous number of people who learned to relish the catabolic foods. In fact, many began to crave fruits and salad vegetables in nearly the same degree that they once sought starchy foods and fats. This lends credence to the theory of nutritionists that man's natural, normal appetites may be trusted and that he, if given the opportunity, would tend to choose a balanced diet.

I am inclined to agree with this view, first because so many of our listeners learn to like and appreciate and really "go for" a balanced diet, and secondly, because in the case of many fatties, this was done in face of the fact that the appetite had once been perverted.

The exact way in which our diet and ideas are used by listeners cannot be fit into any strict pattern. I believe most of them follow the seven-day diet almost to the letter except for foods unobtainable in their locality.

Perhaps it is easier for them to follow the set routine although with a little time and trouble it is easy enough to plan "personal" reducing meals on the catabolic principle which will more nearly suit individual tastes. Some people who have needed to or wanted to take off 25, 30, or 40 pounds have followed our diet strictly for weeks and even months. Many, however, of those who had a great deal of weight to attack have worked out their personal menus by making proper substitutions.

Others have specialized in certain favored reducing meals, using them over and over again. I have no exact figures on how many people have kept their weight down once they have taken it off. I have tried rather diligently to gather such figures but they vary, even with the individual.

Some people will hold their weight down for months and then go on an eating binge or a spree, as they express it. Most of those who do control their weight follow about the system I do—of tackling the problem each day, or almost every day. Some, however, use an alternate system of dieting one day and "letting go" the next day.

Many prefer to eat a reducing breakfast, a reducing lunch, and relax their dietary vigilance at dinner. We can put down no hard or fast rules because each individual is apt to work out what suits him best. When we speak of individuals who have learned to control their weight, we speak of those with whom the fact is accomplished, so however they have achieved it is the right way for them.

We have hundreds of letters from people who have kept their weight under control by simply giving up one or two articles of food to which they had become accustomed or addicted or in which they indulged too liberally.

A number reported that they prevented fat accumulation by eating a "lot of cabbage," many salads, or fruit desserts. Whether this was accomplished by increasing the catabolic processes in the body with a liberal amount of catabolic foods or by replacing fat-adding foods with fat-demolishing foods is only of theoretical interest.

Probably the results come from both factors because, all in all, it must obviously be possible for most overweight people to keep from gaining weight by the simple expedient of adding more catabolic foods to their diet in place of anabolic foods.

Let me point out again that if you should eat a portion of meat which theoretically gives you 150 net calories of fat, you can offset that gain by eating goodly portions of catabolic vegetables.

We may have burst the confines of this chapter with our speculations upon the aftermath of the reducing diet. Lest we sound a bit complacent about our achievements, let us remind ourselves how little we really have accomplished.

As was stated before, we have estimated that there are 16 million overweight adults in this country. If 300,000 people have adopted and used our catabolic system (and I think, considering the number of reducing diet booklets we have sold and the volume of mail on the subject, that would be a fair estimate), even at that figure we have reached less than 2 per cent of those we should reach. So we have a long way to go.

But it is high time now that we come to the most important part of our book, the discussion of the reducing diet itself, so let's go!

CHAPTER TWELVE

"Debble Fat" Is Defeated

Now WE ARE READY to go into the diet itself, which is, of course, the pièce de résistance of our whole reducing plan. Because this diet has almost 90 per cent catabolic efficiency, the three pounds of food it permits you to eat each day should make moderate overweights lose about a pound of fat per day. This is taking all ages, groups, and degrees of obesity as a great general average. Persons considerably overweight will lose more.

That fatty OIL under your skin is going to disappear. Those who fail to take off weight at the expected rate are usually those who fail to carry out the diet to the letter. Sometimes they are people who cheat a bit. Lack of success is often due to a lack of comprehension of the whole principle involved.

For example, a lady went on the diet with her daughter. The daughter, weighing 171 pounds, lost ten pounds in seven days; the mother, who weighed 214, lost only two pounds. Bewildered, the mother wrote us and said that she had followed the diet exactly *except that she had been a heavy starch eater and was afraid to go without bread.* So she ate three pieces of bread a meal, just as had been her usual custom!

Once in a while a dieter does not lose weight the first day. There is a reason. It has to do with the water balance in the body. When fat is oxidized or burned in the body, water is formed. Ordinarily this is eliminated through the skin, the breath, the kidneys, or the intestines. Sometimes it is temporarily held by the tissues. Thus, while the dieter really has burned fat, his loss does not show on the scales. However, it will in a day or two when the water metabolism adjusts itself.

It is even possible apparently to gain weight in this situation. However, such a gain is most temporary. Our body tissues do not get water just from the fluids we drink; they get a considerable amount from the foods we eat. If a person were not eating or drinking, he would make some of the body tissues into water.

Here is a most peculiar chemical fact. A hundred ounces of body fat will yield 107.1 ounces of water. That is because the element of hydrogen in body fat picks oxygen out of the blood to form water. Also, out of 100 ounces of alcohol, the body will get 117.4 ounces of water. That is why people who drink too much alcohol may become waterlogged and flabby. In this strange water metabolism, starches and proteins act differently. A hundred ounces of starch will yield only 55.1 ounces of water while a hundred grams of protein will yield but 41.3 ounces of water.

The ability of the body to make water out of body tissues is a very important physiological fact. Perhaps we can best emphasize it by considering the camel. A camel's hump is composed of fat. Nature has provided it to give him an excellent source of water in case he cannot find any in the desert. One hundred pounds of fat in a camel's hump will give him 107 pounds of water. So Nature, in a sense, concentrates the water for him.

Furthermore, in this involved and intricate process of water metabolism, the deposit of certain tissues in the body adds water to the body content. If you add an ounce of muscle tissue to the body, it requires three ounces of water to bind that protein in the tissues. If you add an ounce of sugar to the body for storage, it will require three ounces of water to complete the transaction.

This is important in problems of weight control. It means that the fellow who exercises and adds muscle to his frame will add four ounces of body weight for every ounce of muscle tissue he builds. The person who eats candy and adds to the sugar stores of the body will add four ounces of weight for every ounce of sugar actually stored.

One point about adding fat to the body is that it results in only a very little change in the water storage as a result. Some very dangerous reducing diets have been formulated because of this fact. For example, when a person begins to eat a considerable amount of fatty foods in place of starchy foods, he loses water from the tissues (dehydrates). Judging by the scales, this appears as a weight loss, but there is a world of difference between dehydration and weight loss, as you will presently see.

Conversely, when a person eats too high a percentage of starches, he becomes waterlogged. That is why people who eat too much starch are apt to have catarrh, swollen nasal membranes, or a flabby condition of the skin. Most important of all, however, is the relation of table salt to water retention.

Of those who fail to lose weight rapidly, some disregard the admonitions about salt and about water drinking at meal time. Their weight loss is diminished considerably because their body water balance cannot adjust properly. Each particle of table salt requires extra water retention in the tissues.

Activities of the digestive system play a great part in maintaining the water balance of the body tissues. Water passes rapidly from the digestive system into the circulatory system and to the body cells, and vice versa.

Many people forget that air and water are essential foods to the body. We could live for thirty days or more without ordinary foods, but we would die within fifteen minutes without air and within a few days without water. Because every tissue in the body is composed of water to a certain extent, our very life hinges upon the body's water balance.

Body fluids are 99 or more per cent water. The bones, which are the hardest of the tissues, are 40 per cent water. The degree of body hydration (proportion of water in the various body tissues) is very important, especially in fluids like the blood. People can have a normal hydration or an abnormal hydration. Thus if some diets or methods of reducing drive water from the body and cause dehydration, the result is a definite disease state.

Dehydration can be responsible for violent toxemias, causes tissues to shrivel and the victim to appear gaunt or haggard, and produces a miserable string of symptoms ranging from headaches to exhaustion. So it is important to avoid dehydration. Any method of reducing which includes this evil is dangerous. And there are dehydrating diets. Some of them, like the high protein diets, have been used; not for long, however. Their ill effects were too readily apparent.

The usual method of dehydration is through the use of purgative salts and violent cathartics. Diarrhea is produced and from one to five or six pounds of water are driven from the body. The unwary victim imagines he has lost weight; he hasn't. He has lost some water and some health, and he soon drinks back the amount of water he has lost.

One of the objections to losing weight by exercise is the fact that exercise is dehydrating, driving sweat through the pores and giving only apparent weight losses—sometimes as high as fifteen pounds in one day. The same objection holds for the steam cabinet, massage, and hot-room methods of weight reduction.

The subject of water balance is almost an endless one. To explain more of the intricate chemistry involved would be burdensome. Suffice to say that our diet does not dehydrate. The three pounds of solid food you eat, with the exception of the proteins, are from 90 to 96 or 97 per cent water. The greedy, exaggerated, distorted fat and sugar metabolism of fat people are sternly disciplined by a high catabolic food intake but, best of all, the water balance of the body is straightened out. Most fatties are waterlogged. Jowls that wibble and wobble, hips that billow and surge, abdomens that undulate soon become firm under the catabolic diet. Watch and see. To a great extent, waterlogging made these portions of the anatomy flabby and floppy. The catabolic diet changes them to solid, natural flesh, not by dehydration but by making the tissue water balance normal.

There is much confusion, even in the minds of dietitians, about calorie values. In the first place, the

calorie about which you were taught in your high
school physics class is a different unit of measurement
from the one used in food chemistry.

The physics calorie is the *small* calorie. The calorie
used in food chemistry is called the *large* calorie. It is
the amount of heat necessary to raise 1000 cubic centi-
meters (approximately one quart) of water 1 degree
Centigrade (1.8 degrees Fahrenheit) in temperature.
That is a lot of heat. Failure to understand the heat
significance of a food calorie is why the person who
believes exercise the royal road to reduction finds it
so difficult to see his error.

Let us look at what this means:

1 large calorie raises 1 quart of water from 0° C. to 1° C.
100 large calories raise 1 quart of water from 0° C. to 100°
     C. (boiling point), or from 32° F. to 212° F.

Thus:

250 large calories raise 1 quart of water from 0° C. to 250°
     C. or from 32° F. to 482° F.—the heat of a hot oven.

And 250 calories can be provided by such foods or
drinks as these:

> 4 ounces of sweet chocolate
> 25 peanuts
> ⅓ cup granulated sugar
> 3½ tablespoons maple syrup
> 2½ cups lager beer
> 2 wineglasses of sherry

I should like to have written "big calorie" wherever the word calorie appears in the text but that might have been confusing. I hope, however, that from now on diet books will give the food calorie its proper meaning of kilogram-calorie rather than gram-calorie, which is the proper name for the small or physics calorie.

The powerful food calorie is entitled to respect. It is certainly not the flyspeck some advertising copy writers make it out to be. Only today, I heard a radio announcer laud buttered pancakes with syrup as a food for people trying to stay slim. One helping contains only 375 calories, he said.

The good Baron von Münchausen would have turned green with envy at that one. Even if the statement were true, 375 calories would supply energy enough for a seven-mile walk at three miles an hour.

If you will remember that the calories contained in food are made less formidable by the cost to the body of *digesting* that food, you can steal a march on Debble Fat. Sugars, syrups, jams, candies, alcohol, and a few other such items have practically no digestive cost. They turn into fat (in us lipophilics) with 100 per cent efficiency. Almost all of them are anabolic.

The qualitative caloric value of certain foods, as far as I can determine, has never been pointed out to laymen, although this is really a more important consideration than sheer number of calories.

Two and three-quarters ounces of potatoes have the same caloric value as one ounce of bread, yet two and three-quarters ounces of potatoes cannot be made into the same amount of fat that one ounce of bread will provide.

The potato calories are harder to get at, or, as we would put it, they have a greater digestive cost. Potatoes are more catabolic than is bread. Hence, bread is more fattening.

Incidentally, potatoes are an excellent food, certainly not deserving of the harsh censure many fat people give them.

I have probably burdened you almost to the breaking point with technical details. I am sorry, but for best results you must understand body fat. And the availability of calories is the pivot upon which a war on fat turns. Remember that just as some foods are more or less catabolic, so others are more or less anabolic. A pint is a pint, but a pint of whisky is more potent than a pint of beer.

We might add a word about the energy value of food calories—with this reservation. As long as our concepts of energy are determined by our knowledge of mechanical engines, we shall never be able to comprehend the miracle of body energy production.

For instance, that little fist-sized organ which you call your heart pumps a gallon of blood per minute through the body while you are sleeping. It pumps five or six gallons per minute when you're running for the 5:15.

Over 500 voluntary and involuntary muscles, all exquisitely turned engines in themselves, work at their special tasks. More messages are sent over your millions of nerve fibers each day than all our telegraph companies handle in a year. Your kidneys receive 600 quarts of blood every twenty-four hours.

Thousands of other functions are performed by the human body daily. The perfection of its conversion of heat into energy defies expression in words.

However, we can give you some basis for an understanding of human energy requirements.

We can reckon that the average human being on a 3000 kilogram-calorie (food calorie) diet possesses one fifth of a potential horsepower per minute, twelve horsepower per hour, 288 horsepower per twenty-four hours (one day).

A fairly good car can be propelled fifteen miles on one gallon of gasoline, which represents 26,505 large calories. That means such a car needs 1767 large calories to run one mile. Yet an average-sized man of 154 pounds obtains enough energy from fifty-one large (or food) calories to walk a mile, and take care of all regular body processes at the same time.

The food calorie is really something!

Perhaps you will find that the calorie values of

certain foods as given in our lists will vary from those given in other lists. Especially in the Meat Substitution Lists (15, 16, 17) you will find calorie values quoted lower than the average. This is because these calorie estimates are for lean meat with all extraneous fat removed.

Generally speaking, variation is unavoidable, as calorie values often vary slightly with the food itself. Foods grown in one section of the country or in certain types of soil may have a little more fat or sugar, vitamins, or minerals, than those grown in other sections or other soils. It should not be forgotten that foods differ in their minutae just as individuals do. Every apple is different from the next; every cabbage is as individual in its own little way as you and I.

But although calorie values, like foods, must vary, they are accurate approximations and invaluable guides.

Cooking reduces the calorie value of vegetables sharply, partly because water replaces the solid matter of the food, and partly because the starch and sugar of vegetables and fruits are soluble. (Note especially that the calorie value of cooked foods such as spaghetti and macaroni is astonishingly lower than that of the raw pastes.)

Practically all the calorie value of vegetables could be destroyed by repeated cooking and washing. This would be a vicious procedure, however, because the

160

the Oriental 7-day quick weight off dier

health-giving vitamins and minerals would also be destroyed.

As is explained in the chapter which deals with foods, vegetables must be quick-cooked, and their valuable pot liquors saved and used. These practices not only preserve important food values but improve the flavor of vegetables.

Each individual food, when metabolized in the body, leaves either an acid-forming or an alkaline residue. And the question of body acidity or alkalinity touches a fundamental basis of existence. The acid-base equilibrium of body fluids, tissues, and structures is of primary significance. It is measured in terms of hydrogen-ion concentration, and the ion is the smallest unit of measurement that can be applied to physical matter. Yet a variance of a few ions in the alkaline state of any tissue in the body is infinitely important to health.

The term *acidosis*, which is employed so often, should not be used in speaking of body tissue acid-base equilibriums. Acidosis covers very special situations in which the alkaline reserve of the body has been completely diminished, such as in the last stages of diabetes. By proper nutrition, a body can be kept on the alkaline side of the hydrogen-ion concentration. When this fails, we call the resulting state an *acidemia* —not acidosis.

This is all important in a consideration of reducing,

for body tissues, being mostly protein and fat, leave an acid ash when broken down. Therefore, during the reducing or catabolic process, as in starvation, an acidemia may develop. That is the harm of a great many reducing diets. They produce not only acidemia but a virtual fat acidosis. The person on such a diet may develop distressing symptoms—and not only feel like the deuce, as the saying goes, but look it as well.

Our seven-day diet is carefully calculated to provide such an excess of alkaline or base ash that it will neutralize roughly two pounds of tissue breakdown a day—a guarantee that you cannot suffer from an acidemia on the diet.

Our diet is not "weakening." In the first place, you get approximately three pounds of solid food a day, and each one of the foods (except those of the protein group) is literally a mine of minerals and vitamins. This is a far cry from "starvation" regimens. Our diet starves only fat.

Since most catabolic foods are bulky, they help fill the dilated stomach that is characteristic of most fat people. As a result, there can be no hunger pains while the stomach is stretched with food.

To provide a feeling of satiety requires much greater quantities of concentrated foods such as pastries, sweets, and breads than of the catabolic fruits and vegetables. The average person eats about six pounds of assorted solid foods a day. The same filling power could be provided with approximately three pounds of the bulkier fruits and vegetables.

The vitamin values of our diet are illustrated by the breakdown of a typical day, on page 229. If you will consult vitamin needs as reckoned by standard authorities, you can see at a glance how amazingly ample the reducing diet is. This fact shows emphatically that a restricted calorie diet can supply enough vitamins.

That fascinating, fantastic field of *allergy*, the understanding of which is increasing every day, promises to be one of the most amazing and important in the healing art. Some of the phenomena of allergy stagger the imagination.

The germ theory of disease, proved by the modest French chemist Pasteur, inaugurated a new era in medicine. The number of diseases now cured and prevented by a knowledge of germs is imposing. Yet the solution of allergy problems gives evidence of becoming equally important and far reaching in the search for health.

Already migraine, eczema, asthma, hay fever, and a considerable number of once-baffling digestive disturbances are being overcome by an understanding of allergy. People who had been plagued with chronic dyspepsia or gas pains for thirty or forty years are now being relieved through the newer knowledge of food sensitivity.

However, space forbids our rambling. Just note this: If you are allergic in any degree whatsoever to any food suggested on our seven-day reducing diet, do not use that food. Substitute another. I will go farther: If you are intolerant of any food, if it does not "sit well," if you have a logical or illogical aversion to it, omit it from the diet.

It has been estimated, by careful studies made at the University of Southern California, that from 50 to 60 per cent of the people are allergic in some degree to a particular food or foods. Probably one person in fifteen is allergic in a degree that produces distressing symptoms.

So, lack of physical well-being while on the diet may mean that you are allergic to one or another of the foods given. Your good sense and good judgment must avoid the pitfalls of allergy. If you meet up with any special difficulty, avail yourself of a physician's tests to determine the offending food.

It was once thought, even by nutritionists, that sufficient calories, sufficient energy, were all that mattered in providing food for man or animals. Then when Justus von Liebig, a food scientist of the last century, illustrated the value of proteins, nutritionists began to take them into consideration. Gradually the importance of minerals dawned upon science, and this factor had to be dealt with.

Thus, the knowledge of food science gradually developed until we now have to provide for almost forty different elements and attributes in planning a balanced diet. These include food minerals, various vitamins, essential amino acids, water balance, bulk, and the acid-alkaline ash qualities.

A balanced diet is one which takes all these (and several more) modifying factors into consideration. It is just as essential for a reducer to have a balanced diet as it is for anyone else, sick or well. It is no great problem to figure out a combination of foods which will starve or dehydrate a few pounds off the body. Almost anyone can think up a reducing diet. However, it requires a trained nutritionist, plus years of careful study and consideration, to formulate a *balanced* reducing diet.

An unbalanced reducing diet must result in harm. Time will prove this—that is why the pineapple-lamb chop diet and its ilk had to fall by the wayside. We human beings will do thoughtless and radical things to take off pounds quickly, but wise Dame Nature's best teachers, Pain and Suffering, soon set us right.

We could devote considerable space to explaining the highly technical considerations involved in creating a safe and efficient reducing diet. Small amounts of starch and sugar are needed to "spare" proteins and to burn fats rapidly.

A certain percentage of starch and sugar is necessary even in a reducing diet to prevent a chemical state called *ketosis*. We have amply provided for this need with adequate fruit in the diet. Besides, body fat is made into sugar when there is a need for it. The hibernating bear taught science this lesson. We have provided enough of the essential fatty acids (linoleic, etc.). They are found in sufficient quantities in quite a few of the foods we give.

There is an important action between the element sodium in table salt and the starch and sugar chemistry of the body, also the body water balance. Please observe the salt restriction closely.

Certain minerals and vitamins must definitely be provided to carry on rapid fat destruction without harm. Careful protein balance must be maintained to prevent destruction of tissues other than fat. It has all been done for you in our seven-day diet, and the chemistry involved need not be your concern. Those of you who wish to go further into the subject may consult any of the standard texts on physiological chemistry.

CHAPTER THIRTEEN

How to Follow the Diet

IN THE FIRST PLACE, get yourself into the proper frame of mind. The diet is not arduous or hard. It is a diet of protective, mineral-vitamin foods which are healing, restorative, and health-bringing.

Practically the same kind of diet is used to treat successfully certain types of heart trouble, gall bladder crises, and other important ailments. The diet regimen is good for you, fat or no fat.

If you wish, the strict seven-day reducing diet can be continued (or used in alternate weeks) until your weight is within 10 per cent of normal. Some people have followed it for weeks and months, practically in its pristine form. As long as there is surplus fat in the body, you can afford to eat foods which will not augment or replenish such a store.

Most dieters, however, make food substitutions in the diet as indicated and allowed. They fit the diet much more to their own taste and food likes or dislikes, and thus make weight reduction a more comfortable process.

Many have chosen three daily menus which they particularly like and used these over and over again. The only caution necessary to give about such a plan is that at least one of those menus should include a glandular meat.

Many, many people, of course, have given enough study to the principles involved in reducing to plan their own menus, using as a basis the general program outlined here.

Essentially, the principle of the diet is one of food substitution; you are substituting low-caloried, catabolic, protective foods for fattening foods. As you are probably aware, most people have no great decided food preferences—they desire only to be "filled up" three times a day. Our diet is filling—try it and see.

Take the trouble to study each day's menu, and if there are foods allowed as substitutes which you prefer to those on any given day of the diet, make your substitutions. Plan to make each day's meals as pleasant and attractive as possible. You will enjoy some agreeable surprises after the first day. When you discover and begin to appreciate the delicate flavor of vegetables (some of which you might never have known), you will *like* the diet, and your way to permanent fat control will be easier, too. Obviously, being a fatty, you have been too partial to the concentrated foods.

Follow the plans and principles of the menus without any deviation. Guard, above all things, the table salt intake. Make no mistake: small amounts of salt are necessary to body health; we must not cut salt intake entirely. But salt demands a very definite percentage of water to be retained in the body. An excess, through its machinations with the water balance, actually helps you to remain fat. So hold down the salt.

Drink no water during the meals. Drink it half an hour before or half an hour after, and drink all you please between meals. If hungry between meals or before bedtime, chew celery. No other food or drink, not even fruit juice, is permitted. After all, you are on a therapeutic diet; you are attempting to accomplish a definite chemical purpose. Discipline is important.

Make absolutely certain of a complete bowel elimination every day. Actually, your entire weight loss is going to be gauged by the type, quantity, and degree of this elimination. Here, too, is a long and involved story. Briefly, any consideration of body nutrition must be linked with the question of waste riddance. The digestive system is not only the larder of the body; it is also the chief channel through which unwanted food residues are expressed. Some breakdown tissues and results of catabolic fat destruction going on in the body are also eliminated.

If a person becomes constipated while on the diet, he will not only fail to lose weight, but will also feel

169

exceedingly miserable. Such a situation is not to be tolerated.

Personally, I do not approve of the use of laxatives and cathartics of a chemical nature. They act by irritation. The use of mineral oil is taboo on the catabolic diet, too, because mineral oil has a tendency to leach Vitamin A from foods, and it interferes with absorption of various food nutriments. Thus, if mineral oil is used, the nutritive value of the diet will be diminished and the intricate mineral and nitrogen chemistry will be upset. Since the diet is swung on very fine balances, we must insist that mineral oil not be used.

Any pill or laxative that causes a watery or diarrheal stool (dehydration) is strictly forbidden. It will upset the delicate water balance which we have taken into careful consideration and so deliberately balanced the diet to maintain.

I approve and even urge the use of the hydrogels. They are aids to elimination which contain no chemical cathartics, and act because they absorb water and provide a soft bulk. A hydrogel added to the diet provides a gentle stimulus to the movements of the digestive system.

Hydrogels are composed of vegetable pentosans. You might ask your doctor to recommend one; use it in conjunction with the diet as a prophylactic against possible constipation.

The diet is not intended to interfere with your daily activities. As a matter of fact, exercise and work will encourage the destruction of fat in your body. Obviously, the more active you are, the more weight you will lose. Many of those who went on the "test" diet aided fat destruction by taking a daily walk, of at least half a mile.

It is easier to reduce in summer, when the skin pores are more active and the heat loss from the body is greater than in cold weather. Two hundred-pound John Smith, who can lose ten pounds in ten August days on the catabolic diet, would probably lose only eight and three-quarters pounds in winter, and nine pounds in the spring or fall.

Because perspiration carries a considerable amount of salt from the body, summer dieters might take a pinch of salt once in a while. This is not a bad plan for any fat person who perspires freely, whether he is on the diet or not, because salt depletion in the body causes most uncomfortable symptoms.

Winter dieters can compensate somewhat for their lack of summer-heat losses by taking, daily, a hot sitting bath. The bath technique is as follows: Run enough hot water into the tub to cover the hips; lean back and rest. Heat will escape from the body, the body thermostat will move up, and your metabolism rate will increase.

171

When swirling currents of air strike the nude skin, the body metabolism increases amazingly. If you will devote twenty minutes in the morning or evening to lolling without clothes in your bedroom (window shades adjusted), you will increase your metabolism rate noticeably and so help your weight reduction.

We have already discussed the problem of food allergies and sensitivity (page 163). If you failed to understand the importance of those passages, please reread them. When the question of food intolerance is involved, the formal diet *must* be modified to suit the individual.

Final Directions: Immediately following these directions, you will find menus for seven days outlined for you. These are the original seven-day reducing diet menus which we gave over the air on the famous reducing party, and printed in our reducing notes.

On pages 188–192 there are twenty substitution lists. Each one of these contains foods which may be substituted safely, one for the other. There are numerous reasons why we have selected these allowable substitutions—chiefly because important vitamin and mineral values have been taken into consideration.

It would be best, although it is not absolutely necessary, to preserve as nearly as possible the allowed calorie values. In other words, if you wish to substitute some other vegetable for the one cup of mashed turnips given in Monday's lunch, you would turn to Substitute List 11. There you find that beets, for example, have a higher calorie value than turnips. It might be best to eat only seven ounces of beets instead of the eight ounces of turnips.

Don't concern yourself too much with this, however, because beets entail a slightly greater digestive load than the turnips. As a result, the increased calorie cost of digestion makes up, in some degree, for the slightly higher calorie value.

While there have been mutterings about the possible evils of saccharin, no harm from its use has ever been demonstrated. Saccharin received a black eye in 1906 when the Food and Drugs Act was passed, and candy makers were enjoined from using it without stating so on the label.

This ruling was not made because of any bad quality in saccharin but simply because to substitute saccharin for sugar is cheating. Many diabetics have used saccharin over long periods of years. During 1914–1918, it was part of the daily diet of most Germans. It is safe to use saccharin for sweetening if you choose. Your druggist can supply it and tell you how to use it.

A pure celery salt may be used in place of ordinary salt for seasoning, or salt substitutes can be purchased at a drug store. The latter are now commonly used, for

173

a salt-free diet is quite often prescribed by doctors in cases of high blood pressure, hardened arteries, kidney disease, allergy, and so on.

Any and all foods suggested can be used either canned or fresh; fresh, of course, are preferable. However, modern canning methods take such exceptional notice of delicate vitamin values that no fear need be felt in using a canned instead of a fresh food. In fact, canned vegetables often have better nutritional values than those purchased in the market, for canneries demand that their produce be lush ripe.

Frozen foods may be used, if desired. They too, because of the care expended in their selection, may be nutritionally better than fruits and vegetables as purchased in the market.

May we remind you that the seven-day diet is really only a spearhead thrust against Debble Fat? It is only relatively important to take off eight pounds in seven days. The big gain is that you learn how to use the catabolic foods. You get the feel of your weapons against fat.

You can settle back, after opening his lines, for a more or less easy-going war on the enemy. You will have Debble Fat on the defensive—or, let us say, where he has you now.

Whenever canned fruits are prepared for any meal on the diet, please wash off all the syrup. Water-packed fruits can be purchased—these are canned without sugar. However, it is more convenient to drain the syrup from those you use and let the rest of the family benefit by the syrup that is left.

A few people have reported that they felt "woozy"— "not good"—for a day or two while on the diet. This may be due to the fact that certain stimulants like coffee, tea, or alcohol are missed. Coffee, tea, and chocolate each contain a drug: caffeine, theine, and theobromine, respectively. The abrupt withdrawal of these produces headaches in some people.

A baker who stayed on the job while following the diet developed feelings of faintness. I suggested that, because he perspired so heavily, his condition might be due to a salt depletion. The guess proved to be right. A pinch of salt followed by a glass of water did away with the symptom.

Some people have a very low sugar content in the blood (technically called a hypoglycemia). For example, diabetics taking insulin may use too much and develop a hypoglycemia. Some reducing diets produce such a state.

Under ordinary circumstances, this could not happen with our diet, as it is rich in fruit and vegetable sugars. However, it is possible that some people with a hypoglycemia might have it aggravated by our low starch diet. They would feel all in or acutely tired. A lump of sugar would restore them.

For the last time, we remind you that while the seven-day reducing diet is very low in calories, its catabolic feature is what causes rapid weight reduction. For example, if you tried to reduce by eating six pieces of bread a day (a very low-caloried diet), you would have very little success.

When you are watching your calories, always remember that it is more important to eat a catabolic food to reduce than simply to eat few calories. It is the catabolic feature that counts.

Let us remind you again that body fat is an oily liquid, not a solid lump. It is a fuel oil which is eradicated by chemical means—food chemistry.

CHAPTER FOURTEEN

The Diet Itself

THROUGHOUT the entire seven days of the reducing diet, it will be best to eat exactly the same *standard* breakfast. This is no particular hardship, for most people are used to the "cup of coffee and some toast" breakfast plan. Especially is this true of fat people, who, strangely enough, eat far less breakfast as a rule than their slimmer friends.

Here is a good breakfast:

juice or whole of 1 small orange	4 oz.	50 cal.
2 halves Bartlett pears (fresh)	4 oz.	50 cal.
1 cup coffee (no sugar)	. .	. .
½ cup skim milk	4 oz.	50 cal.
TOTAL	12 oz.	150 cal.

This breakfast is *only* a suggestion. You may substitute milk for coffee, if you prefer, or even tea—or, for that matter, a coffee substitute. For the orange juice, you may substitute any fruit juice in Substitute List 2. Any fruit in Substitute Lists 1 or 4 may be eaten instead of the pears.

Even though it has been your habit to drink only coffee, with perhaps not even a roll or a piece of toast, you *must* eat some sort of fruit, and eat at least 150 calories, on our reducing plan. In the first place, we want the catabolic action of these fruits, and, equally important, we want the vitamin and mineral values of fruits as well as their alkaline ash.

So plan your own breakfast, if you please, but eat it religiously.

Monday, the First Day*: Good morning. Digestive hygiene, before or after breakfast. How about an air bath? Weigh yourself, after elimination. Remember to watch your salt intake. Drink no water at your meals.

STANDARD BREAKFAST
Don't skip it—remember you have to eat to reduce.

SUBSTITUTION LIST	LUNCHEON	OZ.	CAL.
6, 7, 8	tomato and lettuce salad 1 small tomato 2 ounces lettuce diet dressing (see page 220)	6	32
10, 11	1 cup mashed turnips	8	60
9, 12	⅔ cup string beans	4	20
1, 4	2 peach halves	6	45
	TOTAL	24	157

*Throughout the diet, the calories given for fruit are for

178

SUBSTITUTION LIST	DINNER	OZ.	CAL.
7, 8	watercress and onion salad ½ cup watercress 4 small scallions dressing	4½	36
13, 14, 15	1 lean mutton chop	4	150
10, 12	6 asparagus stalks (6"), dressing	4	20
1, 2, 4	⅔ cup pineapple	4	45
	TOTAL	16½	251

Total calories for day—558
Total amount of food for day—3 lbs., 4½ oz.

Tuesday, the Second Day: Good morning. Again, digestive hygiene? Weigh yourself afterward. An air bath will clear your head. It would be silly to cheat today or to forget about salt and water drinking at meals. Yesterday wasn't half bad, was it? Just note how energetic you will be today.

STANDARD BREAKFAST
It will set you back if you don't eat it.

the fresh variety. Canned varieties have slightly higher calorie values unless washed or water-packed.

SUBSTITUTION LIST	LUNCHEON	OZ.	CAL.
6, 8	cabbage and pimiento salad 1 cup cabbage 2 slices pimiento 1 tablespoon parsley	7	45
16, 18, 19	1 sliced hard-boiled egg	1½	75
7, 10, 11	½ cup carrots	2½	25
1, 2, 4	4 apricot halves	1½	30
	TOTAL	12½	175

SUBSTITUTION LIST	DINNER	OZ.	CAL.
6, 8	shredded radish salad 3 ounces radish 3 ounces lettuce diet dressing	6	25
13, 14	codfish steak filet	4	110
10, 12	⅔ cup spinach	5	18
11, 12	1 cup squash	6	27
3, 5	¾ cup strawberries	3	35
	TOTAL	24	215

Total calories for day—540
Total amount of food for day—3 lbs., ½ oz.

Wednesday, the Third Day: Good morning. Again, how about digestive hygiene? Weigh yourself afterward. Then take your air bath. The diet will be much easier going today. Remember, though, watch your salt intake and drink *no* water at mealtimes.

STANDARD BREAKFAST
Your fruit breakfast helps to alkalinize.

SUBSTITUTION LIST	LUNCHEON	OZ.	CAL.
6, 8	cucumber salad 　1 cucumber (4x2½") 　1 ounce shredded cabbage 　1 scallion 　dressing	6	34
18, 19	cottage cheese and chives	3	86
3, 4, 5	½ cup apple sauce—no sugar	4	60
	TOTAL	13	180

SUBSTITUTION LIST	DINNER	OZ.	CAL.
6, 7, 8	romaine salad 10 leaves romaine dressing	3½	20
10, 11	½ cup boiled onions	2	22
16, 19	beef liver	4	155
9, 12	⅔ cup wax beans	4	20
3, 5	½ cup Queen Anne cherries*	3	35
	TOTAL	16½	252

*Canned, washed.

BEFORE RETIRING	OZ.	CAL.
½ grapefruit (3½" wide)	4	40

Total calories for day—622
Total amount of food for day—2 lbs., 13½ oz.

Thursday, the Fourth Day: Good morning. Daily hygiene? Don't you like your air baths? Now what do the scales say? Swell! Drink no water at your meals.

STANDARD BREAKFAST
Don't skip it—remember you have to eat to reduce.

SUBSTITUTION LIST	LUNCHEON	OZ.	CAL.
6, 7, 8	celery stuffed with cottage cheese 3 stalks celery 1½ ounces cheese	4	66
9, 10	⅔ cup broiled oyster plant	4	45
10, 12	½ cup red cabbage	2	20
1, 2, 4	½ grapefruit (3½" wide)	4	40
	TOTAL	14	171

SUBSTITUTION LIST	DINNER	OZ.	CAL.
6, 7, 8	escarole salad 6 leaves escarole 1 tablespoon dressing	2	15
10, 12	⅓ cup broccoli	3	24
9, 11, 12	⅔ cup sauerkraut	4	30
15, 17	broiled, lean round steak (roast beef)	4	170
3, 5	½ cup cherries*	3	35
	TOTAL	16	274

*Canned, washed.

	OZ.	CAL.
BEFORE RETIRING		
½ grapefruit (3½″ wide)	4	40

Total calories for day—635
Total amount of food for day—2 lbs., 14 oz.

Friday, the Fifth Day: Good morning. Digestive hygiene should be like clockwork by now, the air bath a welcome freedom. So you didn't think it possible to lose weight so fast and pleasantly? You know, too, that you can get along without so much salt. We won't even remind you not to cheat. Do your water drinking between meals, and steer clear of nibbles.

STANDARD BREAKFAST
Don't skip it—remember you have to eat to reduce.

SUBSTITUTION LIST	LUNCHEON	OZ.	CAL.
6, 7	asparagus salad 4 stalks asparagus 1 lettuce leaf 1 scallion diet dressing	3	22
11	1 cup baked cauliflower	4	20
9, 12	½ cup young peas	4	60
9, 11	½ cup carrots	3	30
1, 2	½ grapefruit	4	40
	TOTAL	18	172

SUBSTITUTION LIST	DINNER	OZ.	CAL.
6, 7, 8	tomato stuffed with celery diet dressing	5	30
9, 11	½ cup turnips	4½	30
13, 14	filet of haddock, broiled	4	100
10, 12	¾ cup red cabbage	3	30
1, 4, 5	4 apricot halves	1½	30
	TOTAL	18	220

Total calories for day—542
Total amount of food for day—3 lbs.

Saturday, the Sixth Day: Good morning. Do you appreciate now how important digestive hygiene is? Where do you get all that pep? Well, for one thing, your body is being "charged" with magic minerals and vitamins. You look so much firmer this morning because the water metabolism has by this time adjusted itself. The compliments of friends are pleasing, aren't they? Salt and water intake are still important.

STANDARD BREAKFAST
Don't skip it—remember you have to eat to reduce.

185

SUBSTITUTION LIST	LUNCHEON	OZ.	CAL.
1, 2, 4 (fruit cup)	celery and apple salad 3 stalks celery (6") ½ small apple 1 lettuce leaf	5	44
10, 12	¾ cup mixed beets and leaves	3	45
11, 12	1 cup cooked mushrooms	6	7
3, 4, 5	2 peach halves	6	45
	TOTAL	23	141

SUBSTITUTION LIST	DINNER	OZ.	CAL.
6, 8	raw shredded turnip on lettuce ½ cup turnip 1 lettuce leaf dressing	4	33
9, 11	okra and tomatoes ⅓ cup okra ⅓ cup tomatoes	6	27
15, 16	roast leg of veal	4	145
1, 4	⅔ cup pineapple	4	45
	TOTAL	18	250

Total calories for day—541
Total amount of food for day—3 lbs., 5 oz.

Sunday, the Seventh Day: Good morning. The last day—so are you pleased? Your body cells and your long-abused fat metabolism are, too. Do you appreciate now why 500,000 copies of the diet notes were purchased? More pounds to annihilate? Stay on the diet a few days longer. Start with Monday's meals tomorrow. Rout Debble Fat completely.

STANDARD BREAKFAST
Don't skip it—remember you have to eat to reduce.

SUBSTITUTION LIST	LUNCHEON	OZ.	CAL.
6, 7, 8	tomato and lettuce, diet dressing	4	35
10, 12	1 cup mushrooms	6	7
9, 11	½ cup turnips	4½	30
13, 16, 17	broiled chicken breast	4	155
3, 5	¾ cup strawberries	3	35
	TOTAL	21½	262

SUBSTITUTION LIST	SUPPER	OZ.	CAL.
18, 19	scrambled egg with asparagus 1 egg 3 stalks asparagus	4	90
10, 12	1 cup mixed greens	4	25
1, 2, 4	1 small orange, sliced	4	50
	TOTAL	12	165

BEFORE RETIRING

	OZ.	CAL.
½ grapefruit (3½" wide)	4	40

Total calories for day—617
Total amount of food for day—3 lbs., 1½ oz.

RAW FRUIT SUBSTITUTION LISTS
(Calorie values per 4 ounce serving.)

(1)

Cantaloupe	29
Honeydew	33
Muskmelon	46
Papaya	58
Watermelon	35

(2)

Grapefruit	57
Lemons	51
Limes	60

Oranges	60
Rhubarb	27
Tangerines	57

(3)

Blackberries	68
Blueberries	80
Cranberries	44
Huckleberries	86
Raspberries	57
Strawberries	45

(4)

Apples	72
Apricots	85
Nectarines	84
Peaches	47
Pears	48
Pineapple	50

(5)

Cherries	91
Grapes	85
Kumquats	87
Plums	48
Prunes	69

RAW SALAD AND VEGETABLE SUBSTITUTION LISTS

(Calorie values per 4 ounce serving.)

(6)

Asparagus	26
Cabbage	28
Cauliflower	35
Celery	21
Celery cabbage	16
Cucumbers	20
Radishes	26
Onions	48
Pimiento (red pepper)	55
Tomatoes	26

(8)

Chicory	30
Chives	56
Endive	24
Leeks	30
Lettuce	14

(7)

Beets	54
Carrots	53
Parsley	0
Watercress	36

COOKED VEGETABLE SUBSTITUTION LISTS

(Calorie values per 4 ounce serving.)

(Please note how cooking diminishes calorie value.)

(9)

Beans:	
green, canned	27
string	23
string, canned	23
wax, canned	19
Okra	20
Peppers, green, sweet	23

(10)

Beets	48
Beet greens	26

Broccoli	34	Potatoes, white, boiled	113
Carrot tops	52	Pumpkin	38
Celeriac, cooked	40	Tomatoes	26
Chard	28	Turnips	27
Collards	48		
Dandelion greens	69	**(12)**	
Kale	29	Asparagus	21
Sorrel	10	Cabbage:	
Spinach	14	red	26
		white	19
(11)		Celery	6
Beets	48	Chervil, leaves	79
Carrots	36	Cucumbers	4
Cauliflower	17	Lettuce	6
Eggplant	32	Mushrooms	2
Kohlrabi	17	Radishes, raw	26
Onions	47	Salsify	52
Oyster plant	50	Sauerkraut	28
Parsnips, boiled	57	Squash, average	23

FISH SUBSTITUTION LISTS

(Calorie values per 4 ounce serving.)

(13)		**(14)**	
Clams	100	Abalone	120
Crabmeat	93	Bass	105
Lobster	98	Buffalo	110
Mussels	77	Cod	105
Oysters	57	Flounder	77
Shrimp	116	Frog Legs	75
		Terrapin	135

MEAT SUBSTITUTION LISTS
(Calorie values per 4 ounce serving.)

(15) Muscle

Beef:
 boiled 255
 chopped 165
 roast 185
 steak 175
Ham, baked 175
Mutton chop, lean .. 155
Veal:
 chop, lean 172
 roast leg (fat re-
  moved) 145

(16) Glandular

Beef liver 155
Mutton kidneys 110
Sweetbreads 220

(17) Fowl

Chicken:
 broiled 156
 white meat 167
 roast 210
Guinea hen breast .. 170
Quail 170
Turkey, roast 195

PROTEIN SUBSTITUTION LISTS (for Vegetarians)
(Calorie values per 4 ounce serving.)

(18) Muscle Meat and Fish Substitutes

Beans:
 baked 150
 kidney 122
 lima, green 152
 lima, yellow 160
 soy (average) 170
Peas 145

(19) Glandular Meat Substitutes

Cottage cheese 191
Hen eggs 180
Soy beans (average) . 170

191

CHEATERS' AND PROCRASTINATORS' SUBSTITUTION LISTS
(Calorie values per 4 ounce serving.)

(20)

Instead of midnight suppers
Beef consommé 30
Bouillon 19

Instead of dumplings
Dill pickles 12
Sour pickles 5

Instead of sodas
Lemonade 36
Limeade 36

Instead of beer
Cider 50
Coca-Cola 40

Instead of highballs
Grapefruit juice 50
Plain soda ....

Instead of cocktails
Orange juice 45
Pineapple juice 69

Instead of whiskey
Black coffee 0
 (saccharin)

Instead of puddings
Gelatine with fruit .. 178

Instead of candy
Ginger 68

Instead of between-meal nibbles
Skim milk 47

Instead of seasonings
Seasoning quantity
Chili sauce (1 T.) .. 25
Garlic 0
Onion 0
Parsley 0

CHAPTER FIFTEEN

Help! Help!

WE HAVE now given you the reducing diet, the very same one which 26,000 radio listeners followed in April 1936. I have not dared to make any modification of it, for some people will insist that no other diet could cause them to lose weight.

Of course, that is not true. The catabolic principle involved is what does the reducing. Actually, dozens and dozens of seven-day regimens could be formulated which would cause the average overweight individual to lose a pound or more a day. The substitution lists were compiled with a purpose. We have, in reality, listed the foods enabling you to work out a catabolic diet best suited to your taste and needs. Do take the trouble to do that.

Then lend us a hand, for there is work to be done. The problem of obesity is too important to be attacked with half-hearted resolves born of shame.

I read the *Journal of the American Medical Association* thoroughly every week. My study of articles especially interesting to me gives me reason to believe that, in the opinion of medical leaders, widespread obesity amounts to a public health problem. Doctors are being prompted to consider and treat obesity as the disease it is. The accumulation of burdening, unhealthful pounds is a disease, just as surely as is tooth decay.

Adiposology is the science which treats of adiposis. Adiposis is the excessive accumulation of fat in the body.

The potential benefits to mankind from an organized, deliberate, intelligent war on fat are tremendous. Because medical progress often hinges upon public demand, you and I can be of help. What inroads could be made in the death statistics of these major killers!

DEATHS FROM SPECIFIC DISEASES (U. S. 1936)

Disease	No. of Deaths*	Percentage Excess of Death Rate Among Overweight Men As Compared with That of Normal Weight Men**
Diabetes	30,406	157%
Apoplexy and cerebral hemorrhage	103,560	57
Heart disease (total)	341,350	
organic diseases of heart		51

angina pectoris	17,760	119
acute endocarditis and peri-		
carditis	.....	63
Diseases of the arteries	73,266	65
Acute and chronic nephritis .	106,865	72
All causes**	.....	32
under 45	.....	14
over 45	.....	39

*U. S. Census, 1936. Figures from entire population.
**Louis I. Dublin, *Human Biology* (see footnote on page 37). Note that these ratios are based on examination of selected men, *not* the entire population.

A varying degree of excess mortality is found among overweights from gall-bladder ailments, influenza, and cirrhosis of the liver. Compare the number of deaths caused by disease with the number caused by automobile accidents—about which we raise such a furor:

Automobile accidents 38,089

Today, a portentous new medical specialty is arising: *geratology,* the science of treating ailments and deformities of old age. Adiposology is a handmaiden to this recent division of the healing art, for obesity hastens the onset of, and often delivers the coup de grâce to, diabetes, arteriosclerosis, kidney disease, and others of the stealthy death dealers which exact a yearly toll in the United States of more than half a million lives. It is only too true that the fatty heart of a 40-year-old man may be a 60-year-old heart physiologically.

Straws show which way the wind blows. The serious manner in which medical journals regard obesity argues that one day these publications will encourage the training of specialists to deal with this ailment. Why not? Should the major attack on such a grave problem be left to any stray mortal who happens to take an interest in the subject—for pecuniary or other suspect reasons? The day is not far off when adiposologists will be respected members of the specialist fraternity.

I have already pointed out several ways in which a physician can be of tremendous help to the dieter who wishes to take off pounds our way. There are others.

We often hear the phrase, "Reduce if your health permits." How silly that is! One might just as well say, "Give up smoking if your health permits."

There is no circumstance in which the health of an overweight person will not permit *healthful* weight reduction. It is the manner of this reduction that requires the judgment of a physician. Much harm may be done by ill-considered schemes. Avoidance of these, and observation of personal needs and peculiarities, are not the only ways in which your doctor can be of great assistance.

196

He also plays the rôle of mentor. Having to report to someone every so often while you are reducing is a great help to the morale. If that someone is a doctor, backed by the authority of his profession, the salutary effect is even greater.

You may silence your own "still, small voice" when temptations arise, but silencing your doctor's is a horse of another color. You will be bolstered to resist cheating because the doctor is a conscience you can see and hear. You know that he will scold you in unmistakable language.

Furthermore, when you face your doctor with no pounds gone in spite of the diet, he will soon find out why you failed to reduce. You can delude yourself as to what you ate or what you did not eat, but you don't tell the doctor a fib—not successfully, anyhow.

Most of us are lackadaisical about goals which we set for ourselves. We need a top sergeant around. There is no good reason, for example, why anyone of sufficient intelligence could not obtain the equivalent of a college education just by studying in his own home with the proper books at hand. But the average man or woman finds it easier to attend school, where one's own desires for education are fortified by pressure from those in authority.

Just so does the lone reducer often need a firm hand. Otherwise, he is apt to find himself in the rôles of the

197

judge, jurors, and both lawyers, as well as the defendant before the bar.

We lipophilics require direction and friendly help, encouragement and guidance, when we are reducing. The doctor can add professional understanding and authority to these. The service is worth a good price. And because we pay for his "bossing," we will have respect for his orders. No one values free advice.

Stop a minute to think about our diet. If our concept is correct, an individual who is fat has an unbalanced relationship between the processes of catabolism and anabolism.

The reason we dub ourselves lipophilic is that anabolism is in the saddle. In the healthy adult, anabolism and catabolism should be equal. Anyone who is 5 per cent off balance is going to be either too thin or too fat, in accordance with the way his metabolic pendulum swings.

If a definite amount of catabolic food in the diet can help regulate and condition the metabolic processes which have gone awry, why not benefit from the guidance of a physician who is better able to cope with this problem?

Would it not be much simpler for you to stay fit with diet if a physician were to study you as an individual? He might tell you, "Look here, Jones. You can control your weight perfectly by eating about a pound of catabolic foods a day." The advice would differ, according to your metabolic make-up, but somewhere is your own formula. When you find it, the road to maintenance of normal weight will become Easy Street.

When I eat about two-thirds catabolic to one-third anabolic foods, my weight stays between 174 and 176 pounds. Just 65 per cent of catabolic foods gives me all the leeway I want for eating fattening foods. I can enjoy bread, potatoes, or a piece of chocolate cream cake à la mode if I so desire.

Thus, we have progressed far from the notion that elimination of one or two foods from our menus constitutes a fight against fat. Such a wholly unsatisfactory and inadequate measure is not even a sound blow to the enemy. That kind of sacrifice is made as a self-inflicted penalty for overindulgence.

Surely you can appreciate that the fat person who has taken on too much weight is not helping himself particularly when he fines himself a few potatoes and pieces of bread for having been guilty of this act. Yet his attitude is, "Well, by doing so I took off six pounds in six weeks."

So he did. But in the past ten years, he has lost perhaps 100 pounds in that way—mislaid them is a better word, because they came right back. What he did was to take off six pounds—and gain them back; take off another six—and gain them back.

That's the fatty's favorite game: put off and put on. But he is bound to come out with the short end of the stick because a badly-functioning metabolism *always* works against him. He works against it only sporadically. He will not change his metabolism or cure his functional abnormality. An understanding physician could help him to do so.

I repeat: the behavior of food in the body is a chemical problem which cannot be solved by foregoing a few good-tasting foods.

If, by its patronage, the public encourages physicians to give serious attention to the treatment of obesity, adiposology will soon rise to its rightful rank. Money spent on reducing gadgets and complicated apparatus (which soon rust away in garages and attics) could pay for the services of adiposologists.

Specialists in the hygiene and diseases of children are now doing work of inestimable value, but we did not have pediatricians until an aroused public began to see the need for pediatrics. It saw this need because, not so long ago (1921–1925), 74 out of every 1,000 living babies born in this country died before they reached the age of 1. In 1936, that figure had been reduced to 57 out of every 1,000 live births.

Hygiene, sanitation, and milk control were important

factors in this progress. Proper diet alone has been tremendously influential, but the basic reason for such improvement was that the problem of infant mortality was recognized and an organized campaign begun against it. (We need a frontal attack now on the diseases of old age and the metabolic diseases which afflict adults.)

Much credit for this civilized advance is due to pediatricians. Their publications, hospitals, and activities have given us an expanding and increasingly valuable science. Why could not a similar division of medicine be established for the 16 million fatties who pay heavily in life, health, and happiness for their disability?

Yet it is to be doubted if any millionaire, even one who is overfat, intends to endow an Obesiological Institute. I wish one would—Saint Peter would give him a proper reward. But insurance companies could and should undertake such a charitable program. Stockholders of mutual companies should, in fact, insist upon this course, because every life-policy holder in the United States is helping to foot a big bill for the cost of obesity. The abnormally high death rate of overweight individuals adds much to the cost of your premiums and mine.

If large industrial corporations can draw big dividends from their research departments, what do you suppose the biggest business in the United States (life insurance) could draw from research about a tremendous problem involving human life?

Lately, I have been getting a premium rebate check from my automobile insurance company for safe driving. This plan must result in much more careful driving among thousands of motorists. How about a life insurance premium rebate to the lipophilics who will agree to drive more carefully along life's road? There is a turning-off point on the road to Debble Fat's lair—and the path from there to normality is not so narrow and straight as you might think.

I don't expect my feeble voice to be heard, but if a goodly number of us did some serious urging, insurance companies might take action. Just one properly sponsored, well-staffed, well-equipped institute for the study of obesity would soon transform the orphan science of adiposology from a Topsy that "jes' growed" into a full-fledged science.

A Parting Word: If you who have read this book appreciate that Debble Fat is not an easy-going foe to be joked about and fought with cardboard weapons, our purpose has been accomplished.

Get to know the catabolic foods—remember you cannot run a gasoline motor on diesel oil. Keep a day-to-day record of your weight because the pounds sneak up on you unless you watch them. Treat the low-caloried but noncatabolic foods as good companions. Remember that beguilements such as alcohol and candy are digested without energy cost to your body.

Previously we have emphasized that, from the therapeutic viewpoint, those in the later decades of life can benefit most from weight reduction. But in a larger sense, perking up the catabolic processes of those overfat preadolescent children who are molding for a lifetime their fat and sugar metabolisms is a greater service.

In cases like these, a heavy responsibility falls upon the parents and the family doctor. Why should such abnormal trends be allowed to flourish?

An overfat child is neither "cute" nor amusing. He is an abnormal child whose future physical normality depends upon the judgment of his elders.

It is definitely much easier to train the fat and sugar metabolisms before rather than after the body adjustments of adolescence take place. Let us do all we can for youngsters to save them from our fate. Enlightenment and education are all that is needed.

In closing, let us bow our thanks to all those whose efforts and labors gave us the precious knowledge which we have been privileged to use.

Let us breathe a sigh of regret that other useful

information which might profitably have been written here could not be included.

Let us toast the 26,000 radio listeners whose letters, coöperation, and friendliness gave us a picture of human experience that we needed to write this book.

And to you, my final hope is that this book has interested you in a worthy modern endeavor—that of keeping fit with foods. As Shakespeare wrote:

. . . that such a one, and such a one, were past cure of the things you wot of, unless they keep a very good diet.

—*Measure for Measure,* ACT. II, SCENE I.

Appendix

In the ensuing pages, you will find the calorie values of four-ounce portions of some 600 common foods and dishes.

How to Use the Catabolic Calorie Charts: All the definitely catabolic foods have been set in bold type. Remember please that these are actually *reducing* foods. For example, fresh orange is catabolic because it requires digestive energy to digest the pulp. While fresh orange juice is not fattening, it is definitely not catabolic because no great energy expense is needed to digest it.

Soups, while low-caloried, cannot be considered catabolic because there is no great digestion expense.

Study the chart and commit to memory the catabolic foods. The more you eat of these, the easier it will be to hold down your weight.

In general, you can reckon that any food which has a calorie value of 150 and under, for a four-ounce portion, will not be particularly fattening. The higher the calorie value, the more likely the food is to be fattening.

Please note especially how methods of preparation affect the calorie values of foods. Thus fried eggs are very much higher in calorie value than boiled eggs; creamed eggs even more so.

You will find a few fish, especially the shell fish, in the catabolic class. They are almost the only protein foods in this division. They are doubly useful, for they supply essential proteins and they do not add to the weight.

We have marked milk, acidopholus milk, buttermilk, and skim milk, in spite of the fact that they are, strictly speaking, not catabolic, because they are so useful in a reducing diet. They provide excellent food values.

Purchase a small note book and record in it all the low-caloried meats and fish that you like. Note also the low-caloried foods in other divisions such as fruits, desserts, soups. This will be your personal calorie chart, which will meet your tastes and desires and be a constant guide and reminder.

Please remember particularly that it is the gravies, the tidbits, and the dressings that turn a non-fattening dish into a fattening one.

All figures refer to calorie count per 4 oz. portion

ABALONE, 120
ALLIGATOR PEARS
West Indian, 134
with 2 tbs. French dressing, 194
ALMONDS, 800
chocolate bar, 685
ice cream, 355
macaroons, 550
APPLES, 72
baked, with ½ c. medium cream, 412
butter, 243
dumplings, 312
pie, 317
pie à la mode, 408
pie with cheese, 388
pudding, 378
sauce, canned, 115
tapioca, 138
APRICOTS, fresh, 85
canned, 123
dried, 322
ice, 129
ice cream, 255
pie, meringue, 246
and prune pie, 263
pie, plain, 265
ARROWROOT Flour, 453

ARTICHOKES, 91
drawn butter, 171
Hollandaise sauce, 256
ASPARAGUS, 26
canned, 21
creamed, 160
on 1 slice toast, 225
salad, 160
soup, 71

BACON, broiled, 680
BANANAS, 115
baked, 135
fruit salad, 100
ice cream, 250
w. ½ c. med. cream, 455
BARLEY SOUP
cream of, 138
BEANS
baked, 150
with pork, 160
broad, green, 115
butter, 185
green, canned, 27
kidney, red, canned, 122
lima, green, fresh, 152
yellow, cooked, 160
navy, 414
soup, 120

BISCUITS,
baking powder, 300
with ½ oz. butter, 420
and 2 tsp. jelly, 480
or 2 tsp. marmalade, 500
BLACKBERRIES, 68
w. ½ c. med. cream, 408
juice, 35
preserve, 290
tart, 266
BLUEBERRIES, 80
w. ½ c. med. cream, 420
tart, 266
BOUILLON, 19
BREAD
Boston brown, 280
corn, 330
cracked wheat, 312
date and nut, 318
gluten, 180
graham, 298
pudding, 270
pumpernickel, 258
rye, 312
toast, 432
white, 320
whole wheat, 298
BROCCOLI, cooked, 34
BRUSSELS SPROUTS, canned, 24
BUTTER, 960

BUTTERSCOTCH
sauce, 345
sundae (3 tbs. sauce on ½ gill vanilla ice cream), 270

CABBAGE, raw, 28
Chinese, raw, 21
cooked, 19
w. 4 oz. corn. beef, 340
red, 38
sauerkraut, 31
CAKES
angel food, 298
chocolate, 410
coconut, 397
cup, 441
devil's food, 453
French coffee, 406
fruit, 480
ginger, 381
jellyroll, 410
lady fingers, 421
petit fours, 450
pound, 480
sponge, 440
with ½ gill vanilla ice cream add., 95
CANDY, 446
CANTALOUPE, 29
a la mode, 135
CAPER, 46

MILK, whole*, 85
  acidophilus*, 57
  butter, whole*, 80
  evaporated, 160
  goat, 112
  malted (powder), 525
    chocolate, 480
  skim, 47
  toast, 1 slice, 170
MINCEMEAT, 327
  pie, 334
MUFFINS, 1 egg, 317
MULLIGATAWNY
  soup, 85
MUSHROOMS, raw, 4
  cooked, 2
  creamed, 75
  omelet, 241
  soup, cream of, 80
MUSKMELON, 46
MUSSELS, 77
MUSTARD, 115
MUTTON, lean
  boiled, 200
  chop, broiled, 162
  leg, roasted, 376
  roasted, cold, 443

NECTARINES, 84
NOODLES, uncooked, 440
  soup, 37

NUTS
  almonds, 800
  Brazil, 860
  butternuts, 840
  cashew, 760
  chestnuts, roasted, 576
  hazelnuts, 874
  lichi, 408
  peanuts, 680
    brittle, 500
    butter, 750
  pecans, 912
  pistachio, 780
  walnuts, black, 822
    English, 874

OKRA, cooked, 20
  canned, 20
OLIVES, green, 360
  oil, 1114
  ripe, 301
ONIONS, fresh, 48
  boiled, 47
  creamed, 250
  scallions, 60
  soup, 40
ORANGES, Florida, 60
  ice, 125
  juice, Florida, 45
OXTAIL Soup, 81

*Note: Not catabolic, but should be used.

215

Diet Dressing: Rub a little garlic around the bowl which is to be used. Combine skim milk and lemon juice in proportion for taste desired. To prevent curdling of the milk, add a bit of salt before stirring in the lemon juice. Paprika may be added for color and flavor.

Weights and Measures:

DRY			LIQUID		
3 teaspoons	1 tablespoon		1	fluid oz. .	2 tablespoons
4 tablespoons	... ¼ cup		4	gills	1 pint
8 tablespoons	... ½ cup		2	pints	1 quart
16 tablespoons	.... 1 cup		4	quarts	1 gallon
8 quarts	.... 1 peck		½	pint jar	1 cup
4 pecks	...... 1 bushel		1	quart jar	4 cups
			1	cup (glass) 236 cubic centimeters	
			1	quart 1000 cubic centimeters (approximately)	

GRAMS—OUNCES		GRAMS—CALORIES	
1 ounce ... 30 (28.4) grams		1 gram carbohydrate	4.1 cal.
3.5 ounces .. 100 grams		1 gram protein .. 4.1 cal.	
16 ounces .. 460 grams		1 gram fat ..... 9.3 cal.	
2.2 pounds . 1 kilogram		1 gram alcohol .. 7.0 cal.	

Catabolic Foods Best Eaten Raw:

apples	cucumbers	pears
apricots	dandelion greens	peppers, green or
berries	endive	red (pimento)
cabbage, white	grapes	pineapple
carrots	leeks	plums
celery	lettuce	prunes
celery cabbage	melons	radishes
cherries	onions	sauerkraut
chives	parsley	tomatoes
citrus fruits	peaches	watercress

Catabolic Foods Best Eaten Cooked:

asparagus	chard	oyster plant
beans, string or wax	chervil	parsnips
beet greens	chicory	pumpkin
beets	collards	rhubarb
broccoli	eggplant	salsify
cabbage, red	kale	sorrel
carrot tops	kohlrabi	spinach
cauliflower	mushrooms	squash
celeriac	okra	turnips

How Much Should You Weigh? This vexing question is hedged in with more if's, and's, and but's than a diplomatic protocol. As I pointed out in Chapter 1, your ideal or optimum weight should be determined from several measurements. The soft tissues of the body are hung on the bony framework we call the skeleton. The skeleton determines the desirable type of build and is the basis from which "ideal" weights should be calculated.

The word "normal," commonly used in most weight tables, is misleading when applied to any single individual. Even a competent investigator, using advanced medical methods, can only say that such-and-such a weight is "about right" for the patient being examined.

So-called "normal" weight charts are compiled by taking the average weight of numbers of people who are the same height and age. Thus, 1,000 men, 30 years old and five feet six inches tall, are weighed. The total weight figure may be 130,000 pounds, which is then divided by 1,000 to give an average weight of 130 pounds for this height and age.

Such a result may have no bearing whatsoever on individual cases. It makes no distinctions about types of build or widths of shoulders and hips. As far as you are concerned, that average weight doesn't mean much.

The best way to find out how much you should weigh is to consult a physician. He can make accurate body measurements and correlate them with special weight tables which allow for all kinds of variations.

The tables reproduced here, however, will give you a much better idea of what you should weigh than the ordinary average weight tables. These charts of ideal or optimum weights have been compiled from different sources, all of which are based on consideration of health and the individual bony framework.

As you will notice, a considerable deviation exists between weights which might be ideal for anyone of a given age and height. Thus, a man of 30 who is five feet six inches tall might weigh from 132 to 161 pounds and still be just about right, depending upon his skeleton.

Because of this swing, the first thing you must do before you consult the tables is to determine your particular type of frame and classify yourself as Type 1, Type 2, or Type 3.

Type 1: The person of average, of so-called *normal*, or just-about-right build. What we prefer to call the standard frame (skeleton).

Type 2: The large-boned, *heavy-set*, stocky, large-framed person with short legs, broad hips and shoulders.

Type 3: The *slender*, small-boned, small-framed person with rather narrow hips and shoulders and long legs.

Unless you are *definitely* either Type 2 or 3, consider yourself Type 1.

When you know your frame type, read down that column in the charts for your height in inches and your age in years. From the rough figure given, you can judge whether or not your present weight is approximately correct.

At first, those of you over 30 may be amazed to find

IDEAL WEIGHTS FOR MEN[*]

N=Normal frame (type 1).

Height in Feet and Inches	14			15-20	21-24			25-29			30-34			35-39		
	N	H	L		N	H	L	N	H	L	N	H	L	N	H	L
4' 9"	83	95	70													
4' 10"	86	96	73													
4' 11"	90	103	76		112	134	106	116	138	110	118	140	112	118	140	112
5' 0"	94	106	79		114	136	108	118	140	112	120	142	114	120	142	114
5' 1"	99	113	84		116	138	110	120	142	114	122	144	116	122	144	116
5' 2"	103	116	87		120	140	112	123	143	115	125	145	117	125	145	117
5' 3"	108	124	92		124	144	116	126	146	118	128	148	120	128	148	120
5' 4"	113	127	96		128	148	120	130	150	122	132	152	124	132	152	124
5' 5"	118	135	101	Indeterminate	132	152	123	134	154	125	136	156	127	136	156	127
5' 6"	122	138	104		135	156	127	138	159	130	140	161	132	140	161	132
5' 7"	128	147	109		139	160	130	142	163	133	144	165	135	144	165	135
5' 8"	134	152	114		143	164	133	146	167	136	148	169	138	148	169	138
5' 9"	137	157	117		147	170	137	150	173	140	153	176	143	153	176	143
5' 10"	143	162	122		152	175	140	155	178	143	158	181	146	158	181	146
5' 11"	148	170	127		156	180	144	161	185	149	164	188	152	164	188	152
6' 0"					161	184	148	167	190	154	170	193	157	170	193	157
6' 1"					167	187	153	173	193	159	176	196	162	176	196	162
6' 2"					171	192	157	178	199	164	182	203	168	182	203	168

[*]Undressed. For clothing and shoes, allow 8 pounds.

no allowance made for picking up pounds in the middle years. I have not made such a concession for the good reason that the theory behind it is completely erroneous.

How many overweight men and women sigh sadly at 40 when they remember their trim bodies of ten or

In Pounds, According to Age, Height, and Frame

H=Heavy frame (type 2).   L=Light frame (type 3).

Height in Feet and Inches	AGE GROUPS																
	40–44			45–49			50–54			55–59			60–64			65–69		
	N	H	L	N	H	L	N	H	L	N	H	L	N	H	L	N	H	L
4' 9"																		
4' 10"																		
4' 11"	117	139	112	116	138	112	115	137	111	114	136	110	111	132	107	110	131	106
5' 0"	119	141	114	118	140	114	117	139	113	116	138	112	113	134	109	112	133	108
5' 1"	121	143	116	120	142	116	119	141	115	118	140	114	115	136	111	114	135	110
5' 2"	124	144	117	123	143	117	122	142	116	121	141	115	118	137	112	117	136	111
5' 3"	127	147	120	126	146	120	125	145	119	124	144	118	121	140	115	120	139	114
5' 4"	131	151	124	130	150	124	129	149	123	128	148	122	125	144	119	124	143	118
5' 5"	135	155	127	134	154	127	133	153	126	132	152	125	129	148	122	128	147	121
5' 6"	139	160	132	138	159	132	137	158	131	136	157	130	133	153	127	132	152	126
5' 7"	143	164	135	142	163	135	141	162	134	140	161	133	137	157	130	136	156	129
5' 8"	147	168	138	146	167	138	145	166	137	144	165	136	141	161	133	140	160	132
5' 9"	152	175	143	151	174	143	150	173	142	149	172	141	146	168	138	145	167	137
5' 10"	157	180	146	156	179	146	155	178	145	154	177	144	151	173	141	150	172	140
5' 11"	163	187	152	162	186	152	161	185	151	160	184	150	157	180	147	156	179	146
6' 0"	169	192	157	168	191	157	167	190	156	166	189	155	163	185	152	162	184	151
6' 1"	175	195	162	174	194	162	173	193	161	172	192	160	169	188	157	168	187	156
6' 2"	181	202	168	180	201	168	179	200	167	178	199	166	175	195	163	174	194	162

twelve years ago! Yet their body frames have not changed in those years. Their skeletons are the same size and should not have to carry any extra pounds. The fact that the average person picks up weight after thirty does not make that practice ideal!

Authorities are agreed that the weight which is cor-

IDEAL WEIGHTS FOR WOMEN*

N=Normal frame (type 1).

Height in Feet and Inches	14			15-20	21-24			25-29			30-34			35-39		
	N	H	L		N	H	L	N	H	L	N	H	L	N	H	L
4' 9"	88	101	74		108	121	99	110	123	101	112	125	103	142	125	103
4' 10"	93	104	79		110	123	101	112	125	103	114	127	105	114	127	105
4' 11"	96	110	81		112	125	103	114	127	105	116	129	107	116	129	107
5' 0"	101	114	85		114	127	105	116	129	107	118	131	109	118	131	109
5' 1"	105	120	89		116	128	107	118	130	109	120	132	111	120	132	111
5' 2"	109	123	93		119	133	110	121	135	112	123	137	114	123	137	114
5' 3"	112	128	95		123	134	112	125	136	114	127	138	116	127	138	116
5' 4"	117	132	100		126	141	116	128	143	118	130	145	120	130	145	120
5' 5"	121	139	103	Indeterminate	130	142	119	132	144	111	134	146	123	134	146	123
5' 6"	124	140	106		134	150	123	136	152	125	138	154	127	138	154	127
5' 7"	130	149	111		138	152	127	140	154	129	142	156	131	142	156	131
5' 8"	133	150	114		142	158	131	144	160	133	146	162	135	146	162	135
5' 9"	135	155	115		146	161	134	148	163	136	150	165	138	150	165	138
5' 10"	136	156	116		149	167	138	151	169	140	153	171	142	153	171	142
5' 11"	138	158	118		153	170	141	155	172	143	158	175	146	158	175	146

*Undressed. For clothing and shoes, allow 4 pounds.

rect for age 30 is also correct for age 40. At advancing ages, the weight should actually decrease slightly—not increase—for best health. As a person reaches 45, 50, and older ages, his circulatory and digestive systems benefit by a slight decrease in body weight.

The reverse of this is true for people under 30. Here a few extra pounds may be beneficial. No attempt was made to give weight estimates for youngsters between

In Pounds, According to Age, Height, and Frame

H=Heavy frame (type 2).   L=Light frame (type 3).

Height in Feet and Inches	AGE GROUPS																	
	40–44			45–49			50–54			55–59			60–64			65–69		
	N	H	L	N	H	L	N	H	L	N	H	L	N	H	L	N	H	L
4′ 9″	111	124	103	110	123	103	109	122	102	108	121	101	105	117	98	104	116	97
4′ 10″	113	126	105	112	125	105	111	124	104	110	123	103	107	119	100	106	118	99
4′ 11″	115	128	107	114	127	107	113	126	106	112	125	105	109	121	102	108	120	101
5′ 0″	117	130	109	116	129	109	115	128	108	114	127	107	111	123	104	110	122	103
5′ 1″	119	131	111	118	130	111	117	129	110	116	128	109	113	124	106	112	123	105
5′ 2″	122	136	114	121	135	114	120	134	113	119	133	112	116	129	109	115	128	108
5′ 3″	126	137	116	125	136	116	124	135	115	123	134	114	120	130	111	119	129	110
5′ 4″	129	144	120	128	143	120	127	142	119	126	141	118	123	137	115	122	136	114
5′ 5″	133	145	123	132	144	123	131	143	122	130	142	121	127	138	118	126	137	117
5′ 6″	137	153	127	136	152	127	135	151	126	134	150	125	131	146	122	130	145	121
5′ 7″	141	155	131	140	154	131	139	153	130	138	152	129	135	148	126	134	147	125
5′ 8″	145	161	135	144	160	135	143	159	134	142	158	133	139	154	130	138	153	129
5′ 9″	149	164	138	148	163	138	147	162	137	146	161	136	143	157	133	142	156	132
5′ 10″	152	170	142	151	169	142	150	168	141	149	167	140	146	163	137	145	162	136
5′ 11″	157	174	146	156	173	146	155	172	145	154	171	144	151	167	141	150	166	140

14 and 21. Adolescents developing into adults show such widely different growth curves that it is foolhardy to try to compute ideal figures. A youngster may grow three inches or more in a year, and "fill out" in sporadic spurts. Body framework is still not established. Only an examining physician is competent to decide upon the optimum weight for a given adolescent.

227

Vitamins in a Day's Menu: The reducing diet provides an ample supply of vitamins, as the following table shows.

MENU FOR THURSDAY	VITAMIN UNITS			
	A	B	C	G
Standard Breakfast				
1 small orange	70	32	49	40
2 halves Bartlett pear (fresh)				
1 cup coffee—no sugar				
½ cup skim milk ..	+	++	+?	+++
Total breakfast .	70+	32++	49	40+++
Luncheon				
celery stuffed with cottage cheese				
3 stalks celery ..		+	6	
1½ oz. cottage cheese	60	20		+
⅔ cup broiled oyster plant				
½ cup red cabbage.			4	
½ grapefruit (3½ in. wide)		40	106	80
Total luncheon .	60	60+	116	80+

Dinner
escarole salad

6 leaves escarole.	21,000		11	95
1 tablespoon dressing				
⅓ cup broccoli . . .	258		7	
⅔ cup sauerkraut. .			17	
4 oz. broiled lean round steak . . .	75	100		125
½ cup Queen Anne cherries, W. P. .	450			
Total dinner . . .	21,783	100	35	200

Before Retiring

½ grapefruit (3½ in. wide)		40	106	80
	+	+++		++++
THURSDAY GRAND TOTAL . .	21,913	232	306	420

INDEX

Index

236

CURRENT BEST SELLERS now available
in paper-bound editions

---

* **ONLY IN AMERICA, by Harry Golden**

  A book to restore your faith in the human race. Was $4.00, now only 50¢. Order M5011.

* **THE GREAT IMPOSTOR, by Robert Crichton**

  The amazing careers of Ferdinand Waldo Demara, Jr., the most spectacular impostor of modern times. Now only 50¢. Order M5027.

* **PEOPLE ARE FUNNY, by Art Linkletter**

  A hilarious account of wacky people and events backstage, on stage and out front. By America's most popular M.C., the author of *Kids Say the Darndest Things!* (C330—35¢). New revised and enlarged edition, only 35¢. Order C384.

* **THE SERPENT AND THE STAFF**
  by Frank Yerby

  One of America's most popular authors of historical novels tells of the stormy life of an illegitimate boy who became a famous surgeon. Now only 35¢. Order C352.

* **THE NUN'S STORY, by Kathryn Hulme**

  The great best seller, with a dramatic message for people of every faith, from which the movie starring Audrey Hepburn was made. Was $4.50, now only 50¢. Order GC54.

✶ STRANGERS WHEN WE MEET
by Evan Hunter

"A no-holds-barred account of sin in suburbia!" This is the best-selling novel on which the unforgettable motion picture starring Kirk Douglas and Kim Novak is based. Now only 50¢. Order GC56.

✶ MY SEVERAL WORLDS, by Pearl S. Buck

A wise, tolerant and vital woman, winner of the Nobel Prize and many other awards, presents the personal record of her tremendously exciting life. A Book-of-the-Month Club selection. Now only 50¢. Order GC35.

✶ ANNE FRANK: THE DIARY OF A YOUNG GIRL

The deeply moving story of adolescence that has become a classic of our time. One of the most extraordinary documents to come out of World War II. Now only 35¢. Order C317.

✶ DEAR ABBY, by Abigail Van Buren

A hilarious keyhole glimpse at the most intimate human problems from the famous "Dear Abby" column of advice to the lovelorn. Was $2.95, now only 35¢. Order C356.

✶ *Order them from your bookseller or by sending retail price plus 5¢ per book to:*

MAIL SERVICE DEPT.
Pocket Books, Inc.
1 West 39th Street
New York 18, N.Y.

2-BS(2)

3 BOOKS EVERYONE SHOULD OWN

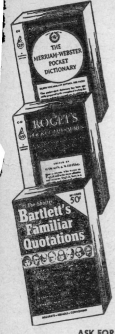

THE MERRIAM-WEBSTER
POCKET DICTIONARY (C-5)

Especially prepared by the recognized leading dictionary makers. Definitions for 25,000 words. Guides to correct spelling and pronunciation (American and British). Synonyms, antonyms, commonly used abbreviations, foreign words and phrases. 512 pages. 35¢

ROGET'S POCKET
THESAURUS (C-13)

A treasury of synonyms and antonyms for everyone who wants to speak and write more effective and more accurate English. Here is a valuable tool to help you enlarge your vocabulary, find the words that express your thoughts most exactly. 512 pages. 35¢

THE SHORTER BARTLETT'S
FAMILIAR QUOTATIONS (M-5002)

More than 10,000 famous quotations from nearly 2,000 authors from Aesop to Eisenhower. Arranged alphabetically by author. Indexed by subject, by author and by key words. 512 pages. 50¢

ASK FOR THEM AT YOUR LOCAL BOOKSELLER.

If he is unable to supply you, use coupon below. With order send retail price plus 5¢ per copy for handling and mailing.

Here's what grateful readers say about this book:

"Not only have I taken off 35 pounds, but I feel so much better and have lost my susceptibility to colds."—Rose M. Schmidt, Cambridge, Mass.

"I lost 27 pounds using your EAT—AND REDUCE. Today is the 52nd day that I've kept my right weight."—Y. V. Katz, Haifa, Israel.

"Took off 40 pounds, but better still, I feel as young and fit as I did 20 years ago."—Bessie Wigger, Noel, Missouri.

"Last September 4 my husband and I celebrated our 26th anniversary and when I saw the snapshots taken that day I realized what my eating had done to me. This anniversary, one year later, I'm down to my normal weight, 81 pounds less than a year ago, thanks to your EAT—AND REDUCE."—Ruth M. Wiley, Whittier, Calif.